Dedication

To Magi for her love and support,
and to my daughter Emma for her strength

G. S. R.

Acknowledgments

I would like to thank Madeleine Morel,
Barbara Lowenstein, and Rodale Press for their
help in hatching and shepherding this idea;
AMR'TA, makers of IBIS, an extraordinary data
base of natural medicine; Dr. Ben Benjamin,
Catherine LeBlanc, Dr. Daren Fan, Loretta Levitz,
Lori Grace, Nancy Lipman, and others who
helped me with their comments and encouragement.
I am also grateful to the many patients who
brought me ideas and inspired me with their own
journeys toward better health.

Contents

"Nature,

time, and patience

are the three

great physicians."

Proverb

Natural Medicine, Back Pain, and You

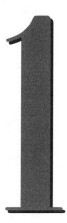

$\mathcal{B}$ack pain affects 80 percent of all Americans. It costs us an estimated $30 billion per year in medical expenses, lost wages, and disability claims, not to mention more than 200,000 surgeries every year and countless human hours of frustration.

Since you're reading this book, chances are that you or someone you love experiences back pain in one form or another, from periodic twinges to persistent aches to paralyzing spasms. Rest assured that you are not alone: Back pain brings more people to a physician every year than any other single condition except the common cold and is the leading cause of absenteeism and lost productivity in the workplace. Unfortunately, modern medicine appears unable to help the majority of back pain sufferers find lasting relief, as the following case history illustrates:

Melissa White,* a 42-year-old lawyer, had been experiencing recurrent back pain since the birth of her second child several years ago. It usually happened suddenly: Melissa would twist or bend the wrong way and feel severe pain in the area beside her sacrum, a pain-prone spot in the lower back between the hip joints known as the sacroiliac joint. For several days, Melissa found herself hardly able to move and would even need a bedpan.

After suffering her second back attack, which lasted for five agonizing days, Melissa visited her doctor, who prescribed a muscle relaxant and a painkiller. Although the medications helped, they also made her feel lethargic and disoriented. After four more years of living with chronic pain and disability, Melissa was referred to an orthopedic surgeon who put her through several different diagnostic procedures. The surgeon found that one of her lower discs was ruptured and suggested that Melissa have surgery to repair it. Melissa chose not to have surgery.

Several more years passed before Melissa decided to explore other options. A colleague recommended a local chiropractor whom she visited shortly thereafter. The doctor took a detailed history of her back pain, including a full description of her pregnancies and deliveries. He also asked general questions about her health, nutrition, and lifestyle. He then examined her back carefully, moving down the head and neck, then slowly palpating along the vertebrae down to the bottom of the back. He felt the way that her hips moved and looked at her feet, moving each ankle, one at a time. Finally, he studied the x-rays that Melissa had brought from the orthopedist she had visited.

Although recognizing that a disc was damaged, the chiropractor felt that what was really causing Melissa's pain was a recurrent strain of the sacroiliac joint. This caused the surrounding tissue to become inflamed so that any motion caused irritation. It also led to spasm of the lower back and buttock muscles, which explained why Melissa experienced pain down into her seat.

The course of therapy the chiropractor prescribed was fourfold: First, he started her on a schedule of chiropractic adjustments of her *spine. Sometimes, she lay on her side while he pushed down on her spine as she rapidly twisted her hip; other times the treatment concentrated on her lower back or even her neck. Melissa was surprised at how easily he was able to find tender, painful spots in her back, even away from her problem area. After the adjustments, the tenderness seemed to disappear. The chiropractor had her apply heat and then ice to the sacroiliac at night.*

The second line of treatment involved visiting an occupational therapist, who helped Melissa learn new ways to move her back while performing her daily activities. She discovered that bending her knees rather than reaching down to pick up her children alleviated a great deal of stress and strain on her back. A new chair for her home office, one that supported her lower back while raising her knees above hip level, allowed her to sit much longer without feeling the ache that had become such a part of her life.

The third part of the treatment occurred after Melissa's back had the chance to heal a bit. The chiropractor then began to show her some slow stretches that would help mobilize the sacroiliac area and keep her back flexible and lithe. He also suggested a daily exercise program that would strengthen her abdominal muscles (weakened since the birth of her second child), work her heart, and help her to release the stress she carried within her.

Finally, her doctor warned her about the dangers of coffee and sugar, which could be contributing to spasms of the back muscles. He also prescribed a nutritional supplement to help cut the inflammation that tended to occur premenstrually.

Eighteen months after her first visit to the chiropractor, Melissa is pain-free. Every six to eight weeks, she receives a chiropractic adjustment, does her stretches every night, and has learned to recognize when she is in danger of straining her back.

*Names have been changed in this and all case histories recounted in this book. Some case histories are composites based on the experiences of several patients interviewed and/or treated in my practice.

A New Look at Back Pain

As discussed above, more people suffer from back pain than any other condition except the common cold. Millions of men and women, just like Melissa, struggle for years to find a way out of the pain that does not involve spending weeks in bed, taking drugs that have adverse side effects, and/or submitting to surgery, all the while never getting much closer to what is causing their pain in the first place.

No doubt you too are hoping to find a way to heal your back while avoiding, as much as possible, time-consuming recuperative periods and costly medical bills. You may also be searching for a way to cope with some of the underlying reasons why your back is causing you pain in the first place. Indeed, this book has been written for one purpose: to offer you options that may well be less expensive, less painful, and more effective than the methods that have failed to alleviate your discomfort in the past.

Most us have been brought up to believe that all things medical can be solved, and solved quickly. As Americans, we take more drugs and undergo more surgery than the population of any other industrialized nation in the world. To be fair, there are times when modern medicine does in fact perform miracles. Without antibiotics, for instance, simple bacteria such as those that cause strep throat or ear infections could race through our bodies unchecked, destroying vital organs along the way. As disruptive and ultimately addictive as painkillers may be, they are also essential to millions of cancer patients, accident victims, and, yes, people in the throes of an acute back spasm. And surgery is often the only way that those with advanced heart disease can survive another day.

At the same time, however, it is apparent that modern medicine tends to look at the human body as a machine, made up of standard, interchangeable parts. Drugs are designed to be taken by millions of people, despite the fact that each person has a unique physiology and chemical makeup. Diagnostic and even surgical techniques are likewise standardized. And it is only recently that the physical impact of stress, depression, and other emotional issues have been included in discussions of the causes and treatment of disease.

A study published by the *New England Journal of Medicine* in July, 1994, for instance, revealed the limitations of high-tech medicine as it relates to back pain. The study focused on the use of the magnetic resonance imaging (MRI) scan to diagnose back pain. Thousands of painful and expensive operations are performed every year based on MRIs that show spinal disc abnormalities (so-called slipped discs). However, this 1994 study showed there to be *no correlation between structural abnormalities and back pain*. Among 98 people without back pain, a full two thirds had spinal abnormalities, including bulging or protruding discs, herniated discs, and degenerated discs. A third of these people had more than one disc abnormality. Yet none of them experienced any symptoms of back pain at all.

Another study done in Norway twenty years ago reinforces this point. One group of people with back problems underwent surgery to remove or repair an abnormal disc; another group with the same type of disc problem was given more conservative treatment, such as bed rest and exercises. Four years later, 80 percent of the people from both groups reported improvement in their conditions. Still another study, published in the *Scandinavian Journal of Medicine*, compared people diagnosed with injuries or diseases of the back, such as degenerative osteoarthritis and spina bifida occulta, with people whose x-rays showed no abnormalities. The scientists found no statistical difference in back pain between these two groups.

This information means what many alternative therapists and others outside of mainstream medicine have been arguing for decades: that too much emphasis is being placed on surgery, drugs, and other high-tech methods of diagnosis and treatment when a more comprehensive and holistic perspective is needed. Indeed, the resolution of back pain simply does not lend itself to the "quick fix" approach generally touted by mainstream medicine and, to be fair, expected by the vast majority of American citizens. Simply taking a pill or submitting to surgery will not, in most cases, relieve backache over the long term.

The Alternative Approach

Alternative medicine, on the other hand, views each human body as a unique entity composed not only of organs and tissues, but of spirit, intellect, and emotion. According to these traditions, health— and a healthy back—can exist only when all of these components work in balance with one another and in coordination with the body's own natural rhythms and cycles. When the body falls into a state of imbalance, natural medicine suggests bringing it back into harmony by feeding it the right foods, stimulating its organs with regular exercise, and providing it with the rest and relaxation it needs to regenerate itself. Natural medicine offers different kinds of therapeutic agents, such as herbs and essential oils, that come directly from nature and are thus meant to help the body heal itself.

Today, more and more people every day are turning to one or more natural methods to guide them through the process of regaining their health. These methods include the approaches outlined later in this chapter and discussed in detail throughout the book—exercise, meditation and relaxation, diet and nutrition, bodywork and massage, chiropractic and osteopathy, Chinese medicine (including acupuncture), Ayurvedic medicine, herbal medicine, aromatherapy, and homeopathy—as well as a host of others. Before you choose to seek care for your problem back outside of the mainstream medical world, however, it might be helpful for you to better understand some of these alternatives.

Why Natural Medicine?

If modern medicine is so advanced, you may ask, why bother to explore other types of healing, especially those that require so much effort on your part, like exercise, eating right, and changing other aspects of your daily life?

To answer that question, ask yourself another one: Have modern medical techniques really solved your back pain problem? Are you one of the millions of Americans who remain in pain, despite spending large quantities of time, energy, and money getting x-rays, undergoing surgery, and/or taking painkillers. Furthermore, you may or may not be aware that natural medicine differs from modern medicine in the following positive ways:

Natural medicine . . .

. . . *is safer than pharmacology and surgery.* Alternative medicine works by helping the body to heal itself, in essence drawing upon the innate wisdom of the body to bring itself back into balance. Drugs, on the other hand, work by either taking over the body's functions or masking the pain that might otherwise help the body protect itself from further harm. The body never fully heals, then, but is merely compelled to operate by a substance coming from outside itself. Moreover, drugs often have side effects—such as the drowsiness and confusion common with many painkillers or the gastric problems related to aspirin—that can be avoided with the use of herbs, oils, and other natural remedies. Surgery, needless to say, is invasive, often painful, and may be disfiguring. If it can be avoided, it should be.

. . . *focuses on the individual, not the condition.* Practitioners of natural medicine recognize that every person with back pain developed the problem under a different set of circumstances. And because no one cause exists for back pain, no one type of therapy will cure it. Alleviating back pain through holistic methods involves not a simple prescription or operation, but a comprehensive plan that recognizes the unique emotional, spiritual, and physical makeup of each individual.

. . . *involves the whole body.* As we'll discuss further in Chapter 3, the spine and back muscles do not work in isolation from the rest of the body, nor do they remain unaffected by emotions, thoughts, or external stressors. While the average orthopedic surgeon concentrates on repairing or removing a disc, a chiropractor, like the one Melissa visited, will treat the whole person—the muscles of the back and the physical and emotional problems discovered far away from the source of pain.

. . . *validates the emotional component of health.* Although it is clear that external stresses and/or emotional upheavals have a direct impact on the body's ability to function in balance and health, Western medicine has had difficulty in finding ways to use this knowledge to prevent or treat disease, especially chronic and endemic conditions like back pain. Not only does natural medicine acknowledge the integral role our emotions play in maintaining the balance we know of as health, but its traditions use emotional factors in creating a comprehensive treatment plan for virtually every disease and condition.

. . . *is preventive as well as therapeutic.* Maintaining the body's natural balanced state is the goal of natural medicine. Those people who visit a chiropractor or osteopath on a regular basis to treat another condition (such as an allergy) are unlikely to ever suffer from back pain caused by a misalignment of the spine because the spine will have been kept in alignment through this treatment. Therefore, natural approaches are truly preventive in that they can maintain function and resolve problems before symptoms appear. An added benefit of seeking natural help for your back condition is that you may well find other health problems disappear along with the pain.

. . . *helps you find the natural rhythm of health.* Your body is a remarkable system of biochemical actions and reactions that allow you to breath, to digest your food, to dream, and to hope. Natural approaches to restoring and maintaining health allow your body to work as nature intended it to, without using man-made and potentially side-effect-ridden pharmaceutical agents.

IS NATURAL MEDICINE FOR YOU?

For the reasons discussed above, you may decide to join Melissa and millions of other Americans and explore one or more natural remedies to restore your body to its former state of health and thus relieve the pain that is disrupting your life. It is important to recognize, however, that to attain true health takes time and commitment. In addition, there are aspects of alternative health care that you may find unfamiliar and, at least at first, uncomfortable. Most forms of alternative therapy, for instance, require that you gain a more intimate knowledge of your body through exercise and massage. You may also have to get used to a practitioner touching your body during examinations and treatment sessions far more than usually occurs with mainstream medicine.

In order to gain the most benefit from natural medicine, you'll also need to learn to truly relax your body and mind. For many people, this experience involves exploring emotional and spiritual issues that may have been ignored or suppressed for many years. Although exciting, and ultimately healthful, such work requires special strength on your part, and support from both professionals and family members.

For the vast majority of people who choose to replace or supplement mainstream treatment with more natural methods, the benefits far outweigh the extra time and commitment necessary. Later in this chapter, we'll outline some of the alternative approaches available to help you solve your back problem. In the meantime, take the following quiz; it may help you sort out some of the questions you may have about alternative medicine and how it might, or might not, fit into your life.

Your Alternative Medicine Quick Quiz

The questions in this quiz focus on four different issues involved in most alternative approaches to health. The four questions in Part A focus on physical aspects, Part B on nutrition, Part C on the emotional aspect of health, and Part D on practical matters. Answer yes or no to these questions, then check the answer guide to find out what you should look for, or look to avoid, when choosing an alternative therapy.

Part A

1a. I can accept being massaged or touched by a qualified practitioner. _____

2a. I am willing to experience some discomfort during my treatment. _____

3a. I am not afraid of needles. _____

4a. I enjoy physical exercise or am willing to make exercise a part of my life. _____

Part B

1b. I am willing to change my diet. ____
2b. I am willing to learn about nutrition. ____
3b. I prepare most of my meals at home. ____
4b. I accept that vitamins and minerals are helpful in treating disease. ____

Part C

1c. I accept that emotions play a role in health and healing. ____
2c. I am willing to explore my feelings. ____
3c. I understand that restoring my body to health will take time and effort. ____
4c. I now include meditation or relaxation routines as part of my daily life or would like to in the future. ____

Part D

1d. I have easy access to one or more alternative practitioners. ____
2d. I have the time and desire to make and keep appointments for alternative treatments. ____
3d. I have some discretionary income to pay for alternative treatments. ____
4d. I can accept alternative therapies that have not been scientifically proven. ____

THE ANSWER GUIDE

Take a look at your answers. Were most of them "yes"? Were there one or more categories in which you answered several questions with a "no"? As you'll see in the guide below, your answers to these questions will help you find the type or types of natural therapy that best suit your personality and needs.

A. The Physical. Many natural approaches to health care require patients to establish a new relationship with their bodies and, in some cases, with their physicians and practitioners. If you dislike being touched by your doctor, then therapies that use physical manipulation as part of their approach may not be for you. Likewise, if you are afraid of needles, then acupuncture may not be the method you'd be most comfortable with, unless you could put your fears aside. Feeling tense while undergoing treatment will work directly against the state of balance that is the goal of natural medicine.

However, because massage, chiropractic, and acupuncture are among the most effective alternative treatments for back pain, it may behoove you to work through some of your fears and aversions with an understanding practitioner. He or she may also be able to help you use the philosophy behind the treatment without forcing you to undergo any form of treatment that makes you feel uncomfortable.

Finally, you will soon have to answer Question 4a with a resounding yes: exercise must become a part of your life if you intend to solve your back pain problem. Stretching and strengthening the muscles of the back, hips, and stomach are first on the agenda. You may also be asked to increase your overall health by adding low-impact aerobic activity in order to maintain a healthy weight and cardiovascular system.

B. The Nutritional. Maintaining a healthy weight by eating the right kinds of food in the right amounts is often a critical factor in the treatment of back pain. Reducing fats, adding fiber, and eliminating sugar and coffee are just some of the dietary modifications you may need to make in order to bring your body back into balance. Furthermore, in susceptible individuals, certain types of food may trigger and/or aggravate the process of inflammation with its swelling and soreness. It will be up to you and the holistic practitioner you choose to work with to sort out these nutritional issues as they apply to you.

As you'll see in Chapter 6, however, you should not feel overwhelmed at the prospect of starting a "diet." Changes in your eating habits can be made relatively slowly, over time, until they become natural, enjoyable habits.

C. The Emotional. Perhaps the most essential difference between mainstream and alternative medicine is the way in which the emotional side of life is considered. To treat your case of back pain, for instance, a holistic practitioner will ask you many questions about your self-esteem, family and professional relationships, and the amount of stress you live under. These issues are as important to mak-

BACK TIP

Carry with Care

If you must carry heavy objects, hold them close to your body at your waist. Avoid shopping bags for groceries; carrying heavy things at arm's length places undue pressure on the lower back. Instead, package groceries in a paper bag and carry it with both arms.

ing an accurate diagnosis and forming an effective treatment plan as the physical shape you are in or the condition of your spinal discs. Because emotional balance is an essential goal of natural medicine, learning to reduce the amount of stress in your life, and learning to better cope with the stress that remains, are integral tasks for anyone interested in solving back pain problems. Such an approach, however, will require you to invest time and energy in an area of your life you may have neglected in the past. Chapter 5 will help you get started.

D. The Practical. Quite apart from the personal factors that may lead you toward a particular form of health care, there are practical matters that you should consider as well. First and foremost is how much access you have to alternative resources. If you have to drive several hours to visit a homeopath or acupuncturist, treating a chronic condition like back pain with these methods may not be possible. Time is another consideration; many alternative therapies require more frequent visits to a practitioner than you may be used to. Acupuncture and chiropractic are particularly time-consuming, for example, as they usually necessitate continued, frequent appointments. Money is another obstacle for some people, since most forms of health insurance do not cover alternative medicine at this time.

Finally, another practical matter for you to consider is your own commitment to the process of natural healing. Many alternative therapies, despite having been practiced in other cultures for centuries, have not been proven according to Western medical standards. (Even many Western drugs have not really been "proven" according to these ideal standards; anyone who takes an aspirin for a headache can attest to that—sometimes it works, sometimes it doesn't.) If you are someone who needs to understand the scientific basis for a therapy, some of these alternatives—homeopathy and Ayurvedic medicine, for instance—may seem too challenging for you at this time.

As you can see, choosing the type of alternative medicine that is best for you may involve thinking about your life, your body, and your spirit in new ways. Because natural remedies are safe and relatively free of side effects, you should feel a certain freedom to experiment with a few different therapies before choosing one. Fortunately, many holistic practitioners either have more than one specialty or are involved in group practices. In the meantime, this book is intended to help you sort through the many available alternative therapies and evaluate which ones may work best for you.

Nine Natural Approaches to Preventing and Relieving Back Pain

Before we outline the various approaches covered in this book, it is important to stress that you must visit a mainstream physician for an evaluation of your back pain. By taking advantage of the benefits of mainstream diagnostic procedures, you'll be able to rule out serious medical disorders such as tumors, infections, and structural problems like osteoporosis and disc injuries that may be at the root of your back pain.

That said, if you're like most people with back pain, modern medicine probably offers little hope of a permanent cure for your condition. The good news is that you may well hold the solution within yourself: Your own body can heal itself if it is given the right ingredients and the right environment to do so.

Our First-II-Tier Alternatives include three methods of self-help: exercise, stress reduction, and diet and nutrition. Except for obtaining permission from a physician or practitioner to start a new exercise program, these are changes you can make on your own.

In addition, you'll learn about six other techniques that may help you in your search for safe and comfortable health care. Each stems from a very different system of thought and, generally speaking, will require much more information for you to master it. But the basic information provided here and in the chapters that follow will help you decide which alternative might suit you best.

FIRST-TIER ALTERNATIVES

Exercise. Since most cases of back pain can be traced to muscle, tendon, and/or ligament injuries, it should come as no surprise that the single best tool for the prevention and relief of back pain centers on stretching and strengthening these tissues. In Chapter 4, we'll show you some of the best exercises for the back as well as outline a general fitness program designed to condition your whole body, including your cardiovascular system, which is responsible for delivering oxygen and essential nutrients to all the cells of your body.

Relaxation and Visualization. The relationship between stress and chronic back pain has been well documented, and Chapter 5 will guide you through several methods designed to help you recognize and then release your own brand of negative stress. These methods include, among others, progressive relaxation exercises, meditation, visualization, and biofeedback.

Diet and Nutrition. Chapter 6 discusses the connection between what we eat and how we feel, specifically food allergies and their impact on the process of inflammation. The principles of finding and treating food reactions are outlined in this chapter, and specific food recommendations, will be identified. Furthermore, a list of the nutritional supplements known to help relieve low-back problems, such as magnesium and vitamin B_6, is provided.

SECOND-TIER ALTERNATIVES

Bodywork and Massage. In Chapter 7, you'll read about several different movement awareness and massage therapies, such as the Alexander Technique and Rolfing, which attempt to both alleviate current pain and realign the body to prevent future back muscle and tendon problems. Some of these therapies require the involvement of a trained professional, others you can learn to do on your own with guidance.

Chiropractic and Osteopathy. Chapter 8 introduces you to two related branches of alternative medicine: chiropractic and osteopathy. According to the theory behind chiropractic therapy, the spine is the wellspring from which the body's innate intelligence is derived. If the vertebrae of the spine are not properly aligned, not only will the back be in pain, but the rest of the body may suffer as well, since the innate intelligence cannot flow to other organs and tissues.

Osteopathy is another system in which adjusting the structure of the body can help improve its function. Osteopaths receive standard physician training (their degree, doctor of osteopathy, or D.O., is equivalent to a doctor of medicine, or M.D.), but their training includes courses on how to adjust the spine and other skeletal structures in order to relieve pain and improve motion and circulation.

Chinese Medicine. Stemming from a centuries-old system of traditional Chinese medicine, acupuncture views health not only as the absence of disease, but also as the ability to maintain a balanced and harmonious internal environment. It is based on the view that humanity is part of a larger creation—the universe itself—and is thus subject to the same laws that govern the stars, the soil, and the sea. Chapter 9 explains this remarkable philosophy and its relevance to the treatment of back pain, outlining the techniques of acupuncture, the basics of Chinese herbal medicine, and offering several exercises known as qi-gong designed to help relieve back pain.

Ayurvedic Medicine. Based on a system developed in India by about the fifth century B.C., Ayurveda, like Chinese medicine, considers health within a universal context. Within the human body, universal forces exist as an energy or life force called prana. Prana provides every human being with the vitality and endurance to live in harmony with the universe, as well as offering the body the power to heal itself. In Chapter 10, you'll see how an Ayurvedic practitioner might look at an individual who complains of back pain and how that person might be treated according to Ayurvedic principles. Such treatment often includes diet, yoga, herbs, and meditation exercises.

   Herbal Medicine and Aromatherapy. Herbal medicine and its cousin aromatherapy use plants and herbs to stimulate the body to return to that state of internal balance we call health by aiding in natural healing. Though herbs are medicines, they are much safer than chemical drugs because they are less potent, more recognizable to the body as natural substances, and are usually used in combinations that minimize side effects. Essential oils used in aromatherapy exude fragrances that have been used as a component of medical treatment for centuries. Derived from plants, each oil has its own distinct odor which stimulates an array of emotional and psychological responses which, in turn, cause certain physical reactions to occur that can help to heal the body. How herbs and oils are used to treat back pain is discussed in Chapter 11.

   Homeopathy. Chapter 12 explores homeopathy and its relationships to back pain. Homeopathy, a system of medicine that attempts to harness the body's own healing power to fight disease and to maintain health, was developed in the early nineteenth century by German scientist Samuel Hahnemann. It is based on the principle that "like cures like." Homeopathic physicians believe that medications should be given, not to counteract the symptoms of illness, as they are in mainstream medicine, but rather to stimulate the body to cure itself. Because back pain involves the swelling and tenderness of inflammation, homeopathic remedies concentrate on helping the body to reverse this process.

Following these chapters on the basics of alternative approaches to back pain, Chapter 13 raises and answers some of the most common questions about alternative medicine and back pain to further guide you in your search for pain relief and general health. In the meantime, Chapter 2 will help you find out if the way you stand, walk, exercise, eat, and deal with stress are contributing to the problems you are having with your back.

"The body

never lies."

Martha Graham

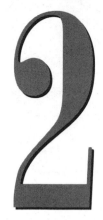

Back Pain:
Assessing and
Reducing Your Risk

𝔐odern medicine has yet to find solutions to the kind of chronic health problems experienced by most Americans today. High-tech diagnostic procedures, sophisticated drugs, and increasingly intricate surgical techniques appear to have made us no less susceptible to such ubiquitous conditions as heart disease and stroke, diabetes and cancer, asthma and arthritis. These chronic conditions, including back pain, are so complex in origin and depend so largely on what we call "lifestyle factors" that standard methods of diagnosis and treatment often fail.

To find out how your lifestyle might be contributing to your particular case of back pain, answer the following questions as honestly and objectively as you can.

Your Lifestyle Factors Quiz

Daily Habits

1. Do you exercise regularly and, if so, have you ever worked with a qualified fitness trainer?
2. Do you tend to slouch?
3. Do you overarch your back?
4. Are you overweight or underweight?
5. Do you take special care with your diet?
6. In what position do you sleep?
7. Is your mattress firm?
8. Do your shoes fit properly?
9. Do you wear shoes with heels higher than 2 inches?
10. How many hours a day do you watch television?
11. Do you smoke cigarettes?

Work Life

12. Does your job require heavy lifting?
13. Do you perform housework or another job that requires constant bending?
14. Do you perform awkward and/or repetitive movements that involve the shoulder, back, hip, or leg muscles?
15. Are you sedentary for many hours every day?
16. Does your job require you to drive a car for long periods of time on a regular basis?

Emotional and Psychological Makeup

17. Do you feel, in general, that you have control over your work and/or home life?
18. Are you prone to angry outbursts?
19. Do thoughts of the future make you feel frightened or anxious?
20. When confronted with change, are you likely to be resistant?
21. Do you consider yourself an optimist or a pessimist?
22. Are you able to make decisions easily?
23. Do you often feel scattered, disorganized, and confused?
24. Do you often feel under pressure you cannot handle?

By answering these 24 questions and reading the paragraphs that follow, you'll gain a better understanding of what might be contributing to your back pain and learn practical tips for reducing or avoiding it altogether in the future. You'll also see that changing your lifestyle—by increasing your activity levels, changing your diet, modifying your work habits, and understanding the effect your emotions have on your health—may be the key to alleviating your back problems.

DAILY HABITS

Question 1: Exercise. On the surface, the "right" answer to Question 1 appears obvious. We all tend to believe that exercise is good for us and that the more we do the better off we'll be. That's the theory anyway. The truth, however, is a little more complicated.

Without question, keeping your body fit is one of the most important factors in maintaining both health in general and the health of your back in particular. All of the muscles of your body—including the hardest working one of all, your heart—need to be kept strong in order for you to remain up and running and for your back to remain free from pain.

Unfortunately, few of us come by fitness naturally. Some people spend their days at work or at home sitting or standing for long periods of time. Others use only a few of their muscles over and over again performing hard labor, such as stooping to pick up a baby hundreds of times every afternoon or heaving heavy cartons on and off the back of a truck all day. In either case, most Americans end up with bodies that are out of kilter with the way nature intended them to be—in balance and proportion, strong and supple from head to toe, with no muscle group neglected and none overworked.

And that's where a regular exercise program comes into the picture. As we'll discuss in depth in Chapter 4, a properly designed and performed exercise routine is the surest route to general health and fitness known to man or woman. By strengthening and toning the muscles of your back, abdomen, and upper body especially, you can find a way out of almost every chronic soft-tissue-related back problem.

However, let us now emphasize the phrase *properly designed and performed* before we continue this discussion. You may be saying to yourself, "But I *do* exercise. Why isn't that helping me get rid of my back pain?" As unfair as it may seem, the exercise you are doing may lie at the heart of your problem. Here are three things to keep in mind when considering whether exercise or the lack of it is contributing to your back pain:

- *Choose an exercise program that's right for you.* Like every other aspect of mental and physical health, exercise is an extremely personal matter. Have you chosen an exercise routine that you enjoy? Does it feel good while you are performing it? If not, it doesn't matter how many miles you run or how much weight you lift. You may very well be doing yourself more harm than good. Your neighbor might have a physique and a mind-set suited to jogging every morning, while your body and mind work in way that yoga or fencing or walking would bring you closer to the state of harmony and balance necessary for health. Pay attention to the way exercise makes your body feel.
- *Consider exercise a process, not an occasional event.* Do you sit all day, Monday through Friday, then become Troy Aikman on the weekends? This "weekend warrior syndrome" is at the root of many a sports-related injury, and more than one case of chronic lower-back pain is due to repeated tiny ligament and tendon tears caused by an overzealous tennis or golf stroke.
- *Use proper form.* Are you certain that you are performing exercises properly? Proper form is the key to deriving the most benefit—at the least risk—from any kind of fitness or exercise program. If you exercise on a regular basis and feel that your exercise is contributing to back pain, you should consider seeing a fitness instructor who can monitor your form. You'll learn more about exercising your back in Chapter 4.

Questions 2 and 3: Posture. Questions 2 and 3 concern perhaps the most fundamental but overlooked aspect of our health: the way we hold our bodies when we are standing. Your mother was right when she told you to "stand up straight." Perpetually allowing your body to stand or sit in a misaligned position—either slouching forward or arching backward—can exact an unpleasant toll on your physical and even your mental well-being, and thus on the health of your back.

Do your shoulders curve forward? If so, you may have found a reason for the chronic back pain that triggered you to buy this book. Slouching creates up to fifteen times as much pressure on your lower back as does standing up straight and also affects how much oxygen you are able to breathe in to feed the muscles and organs of your body.

Do you stand in military posture, with your head and shoulders thrust back and the knees locked? If so, you're not much better off than someone who slouches in terms of the health of your back. The sway in the back that results from what some of us mistakenly believe is "standing straight" puts excessive strain on the spine, the knees, and the shoulders. A protruding stomach, caused by excess fat, by lack of muscle tone, or through pregnancy, may also result in the swayback effect.

Here are a few tips for standing tall: Think of your body as consisting of interlocking blocks that must sit one on top of another in neat order—the head upon the neck and spine, the neck upon the rib cage, the rib cage upon the pelvis, the pelvis upon the thighs, the thighs upon the shins, the shins upon the ankles, the ankles upon the feet. Now, while standing at a mirror in a natural posture, take a look at your own profile. You should be able to draw a straight line starting in front of your ear and moving down through your shoulder, the center of your hip, kneecap, and ankle bone. (Figure 1 should help you get the picture.). If this posture does not come naturally to you, it may help you to practice the *pelvic tilt* in which your buttocks are tucked under your abdomen while you contract your abdominal muscles.

Here are a few other tips for standing, especially if you must stand for long periods of time:

- Shift positions often. Remaining in one position may cause muscle fatigue in both your back and abdomen.

- Rest one foot on something—the rung of a stool or the bottom of a counter should help you keep one foot about six to eight inches off the ground when you are standing or sitting for long periods of time. This is an easy and natural way to maintain the proper pelvic tilt.
- Check your posture often. Readjust your stance whenever necessary to maintain good form.
- Wear comfortable shoes, with low heels. There's nothing like a too-tight pair of shoes to throw off your posture.

Question 4: Body Shape. Are you carrying 10 or more pounds of extra weight? Or are you under the weight that most guidelines have set for someone of your height? Are you pregnant? If you can answer yes to any of these questions related to body shape, you may be at special risk of developing back strain and pain.

You've probably noticed how often we use the word "balance" when the subject of health is raised. This concept is especially important when discussing how body shape relates to the health and fitness of the back. Being too fat, especially if you carry much of the extra weight in your stomach or chest, puts extra strain on your lower back. Your back muscles must work harder in order to hold you upright, and the harder they work, the more vulnerable they are to injury.

On the other hand, being too thin has its risks as well. If you weigh significantly less than what is recommended for your height, it is likely that your muscles are underdeveloped and thus lack the strength to hold your body in alignment.

Women have two specific issues related to body shape and back pain. Women with very large breasts and women who are pregnant are at particularly high risk for back pain, and for largely the same reason. In both cases they are carrying extra weight at the front of their bodies, thereby placing excess strain on their lower backs, the muscles of which are largely responsible for holding the body in alignment.

Here are a few tips for maintaining a healthy body shape: Talk to your physician if you are concerned about your weight. He or she may suggest performing a simple test to determine how much body fat you

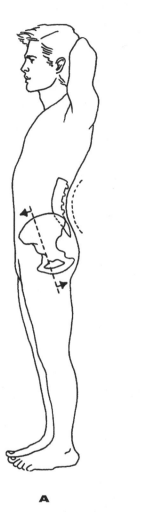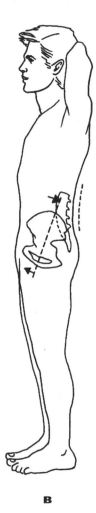

A   B

Pelvic Tilt

*(a) Notice the way that the back is swayed,
the pelvis tilted back, and the knees are locked. This posture often leads to
chronic back pain. (b) Here you see the "pelvic tilt" in action:
The pelvis rotates forward, bringing the spine into alignment
and removing the sway from the back, and the knees are relaxed.
Practice this movement until it comes naturally to you.*

are carrying, as well as outline a diet and exercise plan to bring your body back into balance. If you are a woman with particularly large breasts, make sure you wear a bra that provides enough support, especially while you exercise. If you are pregnant, talk to your obstetrician about your back pain problems and see Chapter 4 for suggestions about exercising safely.

Question 5: Diet. It might be hard to imagine that your diet might have an impact on the health of your back, but there are at least three ways in which it does. First, eating too many or too few calories every day puts you at risk for becoming obese or underweight, which puts the back at special risk for stress and strain.

Second, the process of inflammation, which begins as soon as a muscle, tendon, or ligament is strained or sprained, may be further aggravated by eating certain kinds of food. For example, it has been shown that vegetables of the nightshade family, including eggplant, tomatoes, and peppers among others, may make muscles feel sore and inflamed, especially in people who are allergic or sensitive to these foods.

Third, eating poorly by consuming too much sugar and fat and not enough fiber can make you feel tired, leading to careless posture and exercise habits. Furthermore, eating poorly may contribute to constipation, a definite factor in the development or aggravation of back pain in many individuals. Finally, if you do not consume enough of the appropriate nutrients, you are not providing your body with the ingredients it needs to heal injured tissue or to keep your musculoskeletal system healthy.

In Chapter 6, we'll discuss in some detail how to improve your eating habits to prevent or alleviate back pain. In the meantime, take the time to evaluate your diet by keeping a food diary. Write down every morsel of food you eat, the time you eat it, and the effect, if any, it has on both your emotional moods and your back pain.

Questions 6 and 7: Sleep Patterns. Sleep is an activity none of us should take for granted. While you sleep, your body and mind are restored and rejuvenated. Your tissues and organs have a chance to recover from a long day of digestion and movement, while your brain enjoys a respite from intellectual and emotional stimulation. With too little rest over a long period of time, you run a high risk of injury, disease, and disharmony. Even one night of disrupted sleep can leave you in a state of fatigue that may well result in a nagging, uncomfortable backache.

At the same time, how and where you sleep may directly affect your back muscles. If your mattress is too soft, your spine will come out of alignment and have to rely on the ligaments and muscles to maintain its normal "S" shape. In that case, your back may end up even more fatigued in the morning than it was when you went to bed.

Sleeping on a mattress that is too hard, however, is not the answer either, especially if you sleep on your side. This position forces the curve of your waist to become suspended between your hips and shoulders, forcing your lower back to work hard in an attempt to maintain its alignment.

The position you sleep in is another factor you should consider when assessing your risk for back pain or when attempting to pinpoint its cause. Sleeping flat on your back or flat on your stomach will both result in placing excess pressure on your lower spine.

Here are a few tips for sleeping soundly and safely: Contrary to popular belief, sleeping with a board tucked under your mattress or sleeping on the floor *will not* solve your back pain problems. As discussed above, a too-hard surface can cause injury as quickly as a too-soft one. Most people find that a firm mattress and box spring are all the support that they need.

As for sleeping positions, the fetal position—on your side, legs drawn up to the chest, chin tucked under gently—appears to be the best position for those at risk for or already afflicted with back pain. If you tend to sleep on your back or stomach, try sleeping in the fetal position as close to one edge of the bed as possible, placing a mountain of pillows behind you so that turning over during the night is difficult. That way, you may stay sleeping in the right position.

One other important note: Both mainstream and alternative doctors frequently recommend bed rest to treat back pain. Certainly, a few days of bed rest during the most acute phase of a back attack is necessary in order to relieve muscle spasms and reduce the chance of further injury. However, staying in bed for more than a few days, a week at the most, may do you more harm than good as your muscles become weaker with lack of exercise. If your doctor prescribes more than a week of bed rest for your back injury, make sure you understand his or her reasons for doing so. If you still feel uncomfortable about your treatment, consider seeking a second opinion.

Questions 8 and 9: Footwear. Do your shoes pinch on a regular basis? Are your feet covered with blisters and calluses? If so, you're not alone. Approximately four out of five adults have painful feet, and a large percentage of them also have lower backaches. Is there a relationship? Absolutely. The foot is built to give the musculoskeletal system a stable base on which to rest. If the foot is injured or out of alignment, or if the shoe on the foot does not fit properly, the effects may reach right up through the legs into the spine. Anyone who has had a particularly painful blister or corn on one foot knows what a day of limping can mean to the back: twinges, aches, even a full-blown muscle spasm.

As is true for people with back pain, few of those with foot pain suffer from mechanical or structural problems of the foot. Instead, studies show that ill-fitting shoes are at the root of more than 80 percent of foot problems. By simply changing your shoes to better fit your feet, you will be helping prevent, not only painful foot injuries, but future back problems as well.

Here are a few tips for maintaining healthy feet: The most important things you can do to keep you feet and your lower back healthy include buying and wearing shoes that fit properly.

- Get a good fit. Have an experienced shoe salesperson measure both of your feet using a metal device called the Brannock scale. Always put your full weight on the foot that is being measured. Choose the shoe size that fits the larger foot (most of us have one foot that is slightly larger than the other).
- Never shop for shoes early in the morning because your feet tend to swell as the day progresses.
- Never wear shoes with heels higher than two inches.

- Groom your feet on a regular basis. Clip your toenails, remove calluses, and treat blisters to avoid unnecessary pain.
- Invest in proper athletic footwear. If you jog, walk, or take aerobic classes, you need a sneaker that will support your arches and ankles. Ask a sports therapist and/or an experienced salesperson to help you choose the best athletic shoe.

Question 10: Television Viewing. Do you choose watching television over taking a walk, playing a game of cards, or involving yourself in a hobby? If so, you may be putting your back at risk for pain and strain. One reason is simply that watching television is a sedentary activity. You're sitting on a chair or lying on a sofa, often for hours at a time. If you fail to support your back properly, you may end up with a chronic, nagging backache before you know it.

Even more important, most of us watch television because we think it relaxes us. After a long day, turning on the TV seems like a perfectly passive and peaceful activity. Unfortunately, for many people who watch television for more than one or two hours at a time, just the opposite is true. First, such long-standing, passive activity leads many of us to feel anxious and guilty over "wasting time." We end up restless and troubled rather than relaxed. Second, what we watch may have a strong and negative emotional impact. One study found that heavy television watchers tend to mistrust others and to view themselves as living in a hostile world. Since many of us tend to hold such tension and negativity within our bodies, specifically within the muscles of our lower backs, it should come as no surprise that back pain may be one result of watching too much television.

Here are a few tips for watching television that will be kind to your back: All good things in moderation, as the saying goes, and this applies to television viewing, too.

- Cradle yourself. Make sure your "seat of choice" offers support to your lower back and your neck.
- Adjust your view. If you watch television in bed, place the television at least six feet off the floor.

- Take frequent breaks. Stand up, stretch, walk around.
- Don't overeat. A bag of potato chips consumed during every ball game can lead to five or ten extra pounds every year, which places even more strain and pressure on your back.
- Learn to relax in more active ways. No one denies that watching an evening's worth of television can be relaxing and fun. But if you find yourself glued to the tube every night, you might want to consider finding less passive ways to spend your free time. Join a gym, learn to knit, garden, read a book, spend more time with your spouse and children.

Question 11: Smoking. The hazards of smoking are so well publicized, you'd think you'd know them all by now. But it may come as a surprise to you that cigarette smoking may well be contributing to your case of back pain. There is a great deal of evidence that nicotine, the most potent substance in cigarette smoke, interferes with blood flow to the spine, causing abnormalities in the normal biological functions of the disks.

There's only one tip we give you on smoking: Stop as soon as possible. The American Heart Association and the American Lung Association are just two of the organizations you can contact for advice about how to quit. Do so right away. (See Chapter 14 for more information.)

YOUR WORK LIFE

Questions 12, 13, and 14: Body Movements. These questions concern the way you are required to move your body during what is probably a minimum of 40 hours every week. Performed improperly, those movements may very well lead to debilitating back pain. Back pain accounts for more than 31 percent of all work-related injuries in any given year. Keep this fact in mind when you assess the risk your job may be posing to your health.

Any job that requires heavy lifting or frequent bending will put extra stress on the muscles of the lower back, shoulders, hip flexors, and buttocks. Such jobs can range from endlessly picking up an infant or toddler to heaving objects on and off a truck all day to assembling small factory parts hour after hour. When you lift an object, the discs of the spine become compressed. And the more you bend down or hunch your shoulders, such as over a desk or worktable, the more time the muscles of your lower back and shoulders spend in a state of contraction.

At the same time, performing smaller movements over and over, such as typing on a keyboard or assembling factory parts, may cause injuries to the arms and hands, which in turn will affect the upper back and neck.

Here are a few tips for getting the job done. In a perfect world, no one with lower-back problems would ever have to lift another heavy object. Needless to say, however, you will probably have to use your muscles to lift in the near future. To avoid straining your back while doing so, follow the tips below.

- Use your legs. *Always* bend your knees and use the strength of your thighs and abdomen—not your back—to lift.
- Spread your legs. Stand with your feet about shoulders' width apart with one foot about six inches in front of the other. This position makes it easier to keep your back straight and to maintain your balance.
- Hug your load. Keep the object you're lifting close to your body. If you lift a 10-pound weight with the weight just 14 inches from your body you will be lifting the equivalent of approximately 150 pounds.
- If possible, divide the load equally and use both arms to carry it.
- Don't bend over. Adjust work surfaces so that they are about two inches above elbow level. Hunching over a cutting board in the kitchen or bending over a tool bench can cause extreme lower-back fatigue after just a few hours. Over the long term, such movements can lead to chronic back pain.
- Remember to maintain the pelvic tilt—abdomen taut and buttocks tucked under—at all times.
- If possible, change activities often. Many employers now see the benefit in rotating jobs to reduce both the risks of repetitive strain injuries and worker dissatisfaction.

Questions 15 and 16: Sedentary Job Strain. Anyone who sits for long periods every day—at a desk, on a sofa, or behind the wheel of a car—runs a high risk of developing pain in the lower back. The extra pressure that sitting exerts on your lower back comes from the way the upper body shifts forward, forcing the back muscles to strain in order to hold you upright. If you also slouch or hunch your shoulders, you add to that pressure.

Here are some tips for sitting without pain: The rules for good posture apply to your body when you sit as well as when you stand.

- Watch how you cross your legs. Cross them at the ankles, not across the knees.
- Choose a chair that supports your lower back. For most people who suffer with back pain, a chair with a straight back, with armrests, and with enough depth and width to allow the body to shift works best. The bulge of the chair back should fit right into the small of your back. The seat of the chair should have some padding, but should not give more than a half inch or so when you sit in it.
- Test drive your office chair. Before you choose a chair, sit in it for at least 45 minutes to one hour.
- Don't vegetate. Stand up and move around at least once every half hour.
- Drive upright. When driving, move your car seat forward so that your knees are bent, and support your lower back with a small pillow.

EMOTIONAL LIFESTYLE

Look back at your answers to Questions 17 through 24. They deal with a subject you may be surprised to find raised in a book about back pain: your emotional life. But the truth is, if you do not examine your feelings about yourself and your place in the world around you, you may be missing the very best chance you have to solve your back pain problems.

Do you feel that you have no control over your circumstances at work or at home? Are you afraid of the future? Do you feel angry and resentful much of the time? Do you often prevent yourself from feeling anything at all? If so, you're not alone. The conditions under which we live in today's fast-paced world causes many of us to harbor feelings of anger, frustration, fear, and powerlessness—emotions usually lumped together and referred to as "stress." Many people, unable to recognize or release the stress they feel, "hold" that stress inside their bodies. Some hold stress in the stomach, often leading to gastritis; others develop heart disease.

In Chapter 5, we'll explore in more depth the links between the physical and emotional within your body. We'll also explore the ways in which relaxation and meditation can be used to both gain awareness of your feelings about yourself and your world and to release those feelings from the places in the body—like the back—where they're often stored. In the meantime, start to relieve some of the excess pressure in your life by following these tips for relieving stress:

- Keep an emotional diary. Write down what you were feeling just before and during an episode of back pain to see if there is a pattern that connects your feelings to your physical condition.
- Let it out. If you discover that you're holding in anger or frustration on a regular basis, try to find some healthy outlets, such as exercise or talking with a therapist for that extra emotion.

You've now learned about the many day-to-day activities, habits, and attitudes that may be contributing to your back pain. You may even find that your problems are alleviated when you follow the tips that have been provided in this chapter. More than likely, however, you'll need some further guidance in reaching the goal of physical and emotional balance—the kind of balance that is required to keep your spine and its supporting muscles, ligaments, and tendons healthy and free from pain. Before we address those subjects, however, Chapter 3 will introduce you to your back in a more formal way by showing you its proper anatomy and physiology as well as describing what can go wrong to cause pain.

"Sickness
is felt, but health
not at all."

Thomas Fuller

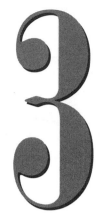

Back Pain:
A Medical Overview

*T*im Peters first experienced what he called a "back spasm"
when he reached down to pick up his infant son one morning. The
pain, he told his doctor, was unlike anything he'd felt before; he was
unable to get out of bed for two days. Bed rest, along with warm
baths and deep breathing exercises recommended to him by his wife's
yoga teacher, appeared to return his back to its normal state of health
within several days, and Tim has, so far, experienced no recurrences.

Karen W., a computer programmer, on the other hand, feels a
steady ache in her lower back almost constantly. During weeks in which
her job keeps her desk-bound, the pain increases dramatically and only
after performing stretching exercises and some aerobic activity does she
feel better. Karen, 42, has had this pain for as long as she can remember.

Tim and Karen represent two sides of the back pain story. In Tim's case, the back attack was an *acute* one: It occurred suddenly and resolved itself quickly with bed rest and relaxation. Karen's condition, on the other hand, is considered *chronic*. It recurs on a regular basis, and no treatment has yet been found to completely cure her problem. A whole host of other cases fall somewhere in between the acute attack and the chronic condition. Some people experience occasional twinges which pass quickly, others expect to feel pain for hours or days after performing a necessary but awkward movement, still others are subject to periodic but debilitating spasms.

Despite these differences in the aspects of back pain, most sufferers, including Tim and Karen, receive the same diagnosis—"muscle strain"—from their physicians, if they receive a definitive diagnosis at all. As the following description shows, the anatomy and physiology of the human back are so complex and interdependent that pinpointing the exact cause of pain is often extraordinarily difficult.

Understanding Your Back

A flexible, gentle "S" formed of bones and cartilage, protecting a bundle of nerve fibers, and held in place by muscles, ligaments, and tendons: That in a nutshell is the *spine,* one of the most elegant mechanical structures in the human body. The spine (also called the *spinal column*) is flexible enough to allow the body to bend, yet is strong enough to support both the head, which weighs about 12 pounds, and the torso, which weighs about 90 to 120 pounds. The spine also functions to protect the body's communication system, composed of the *spinal cord* and its complex of nerves. The nervous system runs to and from the spinal column and every organ and tissue throughout the body.

The spinal column forms the center of the musculoskeletal system. The legs are connected to the spine via the pelvis, the arms via the shoulder girdle, the chest by the ribs, and the head sits atop the spine

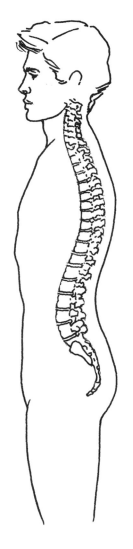

Human Spine

*The bones of the back constitute a complex and beautiful
piece of natural architecture.*

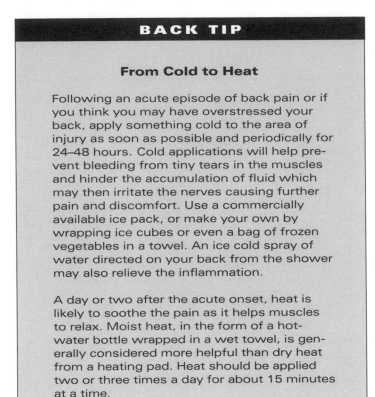

BACK TIP

From Cold to Heat

Following an acute episode of back pain or if you think you may have overstressed your back, apply something cold to the area of injury as soon as possible and periodically for 24–48 hours. Cold applications will help prevent bleeding from tiny tears in the muscles and hinder the accumulation of fluid which may then irritate the nerves causing further pain and discomfort. Use a commercially available ice pack, or make your own by wrapping ice cubes or even a bag of frozen vegetables in a towel. An ice cold spray of water directed on your back from the shower may also relieve the inflammation.

A day or two after the acute onset, heat is likely to soothe the pain as it helps muscles to relax. Moist heat, in the form of a hot-water bottle wrapped in a wet towel, is generally considered more helpful than dry heat from a heating pad. Heat should be applied two or three times a day for about 15 minutes at a time.

itself. In addition, the bones of the spine, pelvis, and chest are supported and moved by many different, interdependent muscles. The hip flexors, the abdominals, the trapezius of the neck and shoulders, and the latissimus dorsi are particularly vital to the flexibility and strength of the back.

In essence, there are three major components of the back—soft tissue (muscles, tendons, and ligaments), bone (vertebrae and joints), and discs (the spongy material in between adjoining vertebrae)—all of which are fed by blood vessels and nerves that flow in and out of the spine. Back pain may result when one or more of these components are malformed, injured, or in any other way compromised.

However, in searching for the cause of back pain, we must never lose sight of the fact—as modern medicine often does—that no one system of the body, including the musculoskeletal system, works in isolation. In fact, the essential difference between mainstream and holistic medicine hinges on this point. To target only the vertebrae or only the muscles when attempting to find a cause for pain is ultimately shortsighted. To find a solution to back pain—and, indeed, to all forms of human disease—we must consider the body in its entirety. We must see the patterns and relationships among systems and tissues and emotions and energy throughout the human form.

Following are descriptions of the various components of the back, as well explanations of some of the conditions and problems that modern medical practitioners consider to be likely causes of back pain. Again, it must be emphasized little proof exists that any of the conditions you'll read about below under "What Can Go Wrong" is a discrete cause of back pain. Nevertheless, it may be helpful for you to read this carefully in order to better understand your own physiology and anatomy and, perhaps, to interpret your mainstream physician's diagnosis more accurately.

Muscles, Tendons, and Ligaments

Together known as soft tissue, the muscles, tendons, and ligaments of the back are quite complex. First, there are the specific muscles that stabilize and sheathe the spinal column. These muscles interact directly with many of the body's other major muscle groups to move the body in any number of ways: bending, lifting, twisting, and walking, to name just a few. Large muscles at the back of the neck provide extension and support, while smaller muscles at the front and sides of the spine allow the spine to rotate and flex. In the lower back, the two main muscle groups are the *erector spinae* muscles, which run down the back, and the *psoas* and abdominal muscles, which support the back from the front.

Ligaments are tough, elastic bands of tissue that connect bones to each other and bind joints, helping to support the vertebrae and to keep the discs between the vertebrae in place. Tendons, on the other hand, are fibrous cords connecting bones to muscles. Covering all soft tissue is a specialized fibrous layer of tissue called *fascia*. Fascia can be likened to the walls of a house or office. It divides the muscle groups and compartments of the body, and houses within it the blood vessels, nerves, and other methods of communication between the various parts of the body. The planes of fascia within the body, which may conduct electrical and other energy movements, could hold the key to the success of acupuncture in treating back pain (see Chapter 9).

WHAT CAN GO WRONG

Muscle Fatigue and Overuse. Sometimes known as *back strain,* muscle fatigue is one of the most common causes of back pain. It can be caused by a specific motion or activity, single or repeated, or may result from chronic poor posture. Emotional stress may cause back and shoulder muscles to become chronically contracted, causing extreme fatigue and achiness. Such contracture also blocks the blood supply to and from the muscles, which prevents the proper removal of waste products from the tissues.

Back muscles often become strained because of conditions that are present in other parts of the body. Sagging abdominal muscles, for instance, place enormous extra pressure on the spine. Overly tight hip flexors, the muscles that work to raise the thigh toward the chest, will tilt the whole pelvis backward to create a swayback, which also may lead to discomfort.

Injury of Muscles, Tendons, or Ligaments. Injury to soft tissue involves the tearing of some of the fibers of these tissues. Tearing may occur due to an acute injury or because the process of inflammation that occurs after injury prevents proper healing. Injuries may also involve small bleeding into the muscle or tendon, causing swelling and achiness. Muscles or tendons may also lose function because scar tissue has formed in the injured structure.

Back Spasm. Defined as an involuntary, convulsive contraction

of muscle fibers, a muscle spasm is thought to occur in order to prevent you from moving in a way that will further injure them. The pain
is intense and, usually, completely debilitating until the muscles relax
once again. Muscles may also be in chronic spasm caused by stress
and poor posture.

Myofascial Pain. Also called myofascitis or myofascial syndrome, this condition involves the inflammation and irritation of the
muscles and fascial covering. This inflammation causes pain both
locally and in other parts of the body (called "referred pain"). The
local sites of injury or inflammation are called sometimes called "trigger points" because they may evoke pain or soreness in the skin and
soft tissues at a distance from the point of injury. Myofascial syndrome may also restrict motion and, sometimes, cause changes in sensation including temperature and skin sensitivity.

Fibromyalgia. Although not universally recognized, fibromyalgia is a syndrome characterized by chronic pain in specific areas of
muscle groups in the back and elsewhere, as well as fatigue, sleep
problems, and other systemic conditions.

Bones

The spinal column permits the torso to bend, turn, and twist, supports the head, and protects the spinal cord and the bundle of nerve
fibers that connect the brain and the body. It consists of 24 bones
known as the *vertebrae* plus the *sacrum* (the bone between the lowest
vertebrae and the tailbone) and the *coccyx* (or tailbone). The spine has
five sections: seven cervical vertebrae, which link downward from the
skull to the shoulders; 12 thoracic vertebrae, which run downward
from the shoulders to the end of the rib cage; the lumbar vertebrae,
which extend from below the ribs to the hips; then the sacrum and the
coccyx. The bones of a healthy lower back are so strong that they are
able to support up to several hundred pounds per square inch.

On either side of each vertebra are four bony protrusions called the *articular processes*. Two articular processes are located at the top of each vertebra and two near its base. The two upper processes of one vertebra join with the two lower processes of its upstairs neighbor. The resulting structure is called a *facet joint*. Facet joints are capped with smooth cartilage that allows each vertebra to move smoothly against its partner and are encased within a fibrous capsule that prevents the two facets from separating. Facet joints lend suppleness and flexibility to the spinal column.

WHAT CAN GO WRONG

Osteoporosis. Defined as a decrease in bone density due to a loss of minerals such as calcium, magnesium, and potassium, osteoporosis results in the malformation of bone. As these minerals are lost, the bones of the spine become fragile and collapse one on top of the other. In fact, an individual with a severe case of osteoporosis may lose as many as 7 or 8 inches of height over time.

Joint Inflammation. Arthritis is a general term for more than 100 different diseases with one common symptom: pain and stiffness in the joints of the body, including the joints of the spine, caused by inflammation and the wearing away of a joint. *Osteoarthritis,* also known as spondylitis, is a common side effect of the aging process. Studies have shown that osteoarthritis is present in nearly all individuals over the age of 75, though not all experience back pain as a result. There are other arthritic conditions that may affect the back, including *rheumatoid arthritis* (the second most common form of arthritis), *Reiter's syndrome* (a disease affecting only men and involving systemic inflammation and diarrhea) and *ankylosing spondylitis* (a condition in which the bone fuses over a joint).

Structural Abnormalities of the Spinal Column. Scoliosis, or a sideways curvature of the lumbar spine, is a common condition that affects about 12 percent of the population. Usually, the curvature is so slight that it causes no discomfort and goes undiagnosed; only about 2 percent of people with scoliosis require any treatment at all. (Since severe scoliosis is usually diagnosed in childhood, it is rather unlikely that your back pain can be linked to this condition.) Two related conditions, *lordosis,* which involves an abnormal curving forward of the spine, and *kyphosis,* humping of the thoracic spine (often due to rickets or tuberculosis), are relatively rare conditions that may also result in back pain if not corrected.

Misalignment of the Vertebrae and Facet Joints. The vertebrae and facet joints may become misaligned and thus cause muscle spasms resulting from the incumbent stress on ligaments and joints. Facet joints may become worn over time through osteoporosis or through an accident or chronic poor posture. In addition, the ligaments holding the joints in alignment may become shortened through the aging process or with the formation of scar tissue after an injury. Once shortened, they can cause the joints to come out of alignment.

The sacroiliac joint, which connects the fused vertebrae called the sacrum to the two large bones of the pelvis (called the ilia), is particularly vulnerable to injury and strain. This joint, located just above the hip, is held together not by muscles but by strong ligaments, and thus has a relatively limited range of motion. Nevertheless, its position marks it as the "shock absorber" for the other tissues of the back. If postural abnormalities, muscle tension, abnormal leg length, or damaging repetitive movements cause the sacroiliac joint to lose even more of its mobility, back pain is often the result.

Discs

Considered to be the spine's shock absorbers, discs are the cushioning pads between adjoining vertebrae. Each disc is composed of an outer section of tough fibrous layers and an inner section of pulpy, semiliquid jellylike material. The discs are thickest in the lower back (lumbar region) and thinnest in the thoracic or chest area.

WHAT CAN GO WRONG

Herniated Discs. Discs can become injured very easily. Incorrect posture combined with weak muscles, damaged or overstretched ligaments, and bone degeneration can put many extra pounds of damaging pressure on the discs. This pressure may cause one or more discs to *herniate,* or protrude between the spinal bones. Herniated discs often occur in the lumbar area of the spine, which tends to take the brunt of daily physical and emotional stress. A common symptom of herniated discs is the intense pain of sciatica—caused by the misaligned disc pressing against the sciatic nerve.

Ruptured discs. Should the pressure prove too great over the short or the long term, the disc may *rupture.* When it ruptures, the disc may lose its semiliquid central portion causing the space between the vertebrae to become more narrow and the spine less stable. Disc rupture is especially common during pregnancy, when extra abdominal weight causes pressure on the discs. Herniated and ruptured discs account for a very small proportion of back pain cases, perhaps as few as 5 to 10 percent of all cases.

Nerves

Within the spinal column, encased within the bony vertebrae of your back, rests the spinal cord: a cluster of 31 pairs of nerves that branch out from openings in the vertebrae to the organs and tissues in the rest of the body. The brain sends and receives virtually all of its messages about the world inside and outside the body through the peripheral nervous system, a system that passes stimuli along the nerve pathways in the body to the spinal cord and finally to the brain (the brain and spinal cord are together known as the central nervous system).

The thickest nerves of the body, the sciatic nerves, emerge from between vertebrae in the lumbar region of the spine near the hip and beneath the gluteus maximus muscle. They run down the back of each thigh and then divide in two just above the knee. One of these branches runs down the front of the shin into the big toe, the other branch divides again, running down the back of the leg to the heel.

WHAT CAN GO WRONG

Pinched Nerves. Pressure on nerves, whether from discs or impingement of bone, may case pain, numbness, loss of muscle mass in the legs, and other problems. Because of its position and size, the sciatic nerve is particularly vulnerable to injury due to disc herniation, a certain type of hip dislocation, or pressure from the uterus during pregnancy. The pain that ensues, called *sciatica,* tends to involve shooting pain up and down the leg and in the hip region.

The Mind-Body Connection

Without question, the mechanical failures described above may, and often do, contribute to the development of back pain. But muscles, bones, discs, and nerves do not function in isolation; the human body is not a machine, driven by some kind of objective internal engine. Instead, the emotions we feel and the thoughts we think have a dramatic effect on the way our bodies work. In particular, the amount of stress under which we live, and how we react to that stress, may play a significant role in the development of back pain. Some of the theories about this connection are described below.

Tension Myositis Syndrome. According to Dr. John Sarno in his landmark book, *Mind Over Back Pain,* tension leads to a physical reaction involving the muscles and nerves of the neck, shoulders, and back. Over time, tension constricts the blood vessels feeding the involved muscles, and the blood deprivation that results leads to muscle spasm and nerve pain.

Furthermore, Dr. Sarno posits, pain produces fear and anxiety—in essence, more tension—in those who suffer with it. This increased stress and tension only add to the original pain, creating, in essence, a vicious cycle that can only be relieved by releasing and/or alleviating tension through exercise and relaxation strategies.

Trigger Points. A related theory postulates that certain muscles, tendons, and ligaments become veritable storehouses of tension and negative emotion, and thus of pain and stiffness. These trigger points, often located in the muscles of the neck and lower back, not only are locally tender and sore, but can also radiate pain throughout an entire region or trigger pain in another part of the body altogether.

Diagnosing the Cause of Back Pain

As you can see, the back is a complex structure directly related to every other part of your body. When something is wrong with any part of your body—from a chest cold to a broken wrist—the resulting discomfort is likely to affect your back as well. That's why the attempts by many modern medicine practitioners to restrict the cause of back pain to the structures of the back itself is often futile. Nevertheless, it is likely that you have visited, or will visit, a physician hoping to obtain a diagnosis. This section will provide information about what such a diagnostic procedure might be like.

More than 80 percent of all back pain sufferers *will never know the exact cause of their discomfort.* In fact, pinpointing what, within the structure of the back, shoulder, legs, feet, or your state of mind, might trigger aches, pains, and spasms is often impossible. Not only is the back's anatomy extremely complex, its physiology is dynamic, which means that to understand how the back works or what might go wrong to cause pain, we must study the back in motion. Unfortunately, the techniques modern medicine uses—and which are quickly outlined here—such as x-rays, CT scans, and MRIs, are designed to examine tissue only when it is still and static.

Although these tools may be able to locate an injury to a specific muscle or muscles, they cannot identify the *pattern* of movement, involving the entire back, that contributes to that injury over time. Neither can diagnostic equipment measure the amount of tension and stress carried in the muscles of the back or whether the person with back pain has been feeding his or her body enough of the proper nutrients. Only by examining all of these issues can a practitioner make a reasonable, if still highly subjective, diagnosis of back pain. If back pain is so difficult to diagnose, and if the vast majority can be chalked up to muscle strain, why should anyone choose to see a mainstream doctor at all? Without alarming you unduly, there are some serious medical problems that have chronic or acute back pain as one of the symptoms—such as viral and bacterial infections, certain cancers, and even heart attacks. It is important for you and your doctor to rule out those conditions, especially if you are running a fever or have other symptoms of illness at the same time as you experience back pain.

An examination by a mainstream physician is likely to include the following components:

History. Without question, the very best diagnostic tool for back pain is a thorough medical history. Whether you visit a mainstream physician or someone who specializes in one of the alternative treatments discussed later, you will probably find that a great deal of time during your first appointment is given over to details about your personal and professional life. A good doctor will inquire about aspects of your habits and lifestyle that may have an impact on the health of your back, including the kind of work you do, your eating and drinking habits, and your emotional state.

In fact, your doctor is likely to ask you some or all of the questions listed below. Think about how you'll answer them now. The more accurate you can be about your pain and what *you* think may be causing it, the closer your doctor can get to a realistic diagnosis and treatment plan.

Things to Think About
before You See Your Doctor

1. When is the first time you remember having back pain?
2. How did the pain first start?
3. Is the pain sharp or dull?
4. Where exactly do you feel the pain?

5. Does the pain extend down into your legs? How far?
6. Do you know what causes your back pain?
7. What makes the pain get worse?
8. What makes the pain go away?
9. Does the pain feel worse when you sit or stand?
10. What past medical treatment have you had?
11. Do you have any other health problems or injuries?
12. Do you smoke?
13. Do you drink alcohol? If so, how much per day?
14. Are you currently taking drugs (either prescription medication or illegal substances)?
15. Does your back problem affect your ability to work?
16. Do you feel under particular stress at work or at home?

After you and your doctor sort through these issues, as well as discuss your past medical history, he or she is likely to begin the physical examination.

Physical Examination. The course the physical part of the exam takes will depend largely upon what the doctor or practitioner has discovered about your condition through the medical history. You'll probably be asked to move in several different ways, bending forward and backward, standing on your toes and on the back of the heels, raising a straight leg perpendicular to the body, and so forth. This will help the practitioner discover which muscles and/or discs might be involved. Your knee and ankle reflexes may be checked to assess nerve function. The doctor may also test the strength of certain of your muscle groups, as well as measure the range of motion of joints in your back, hips, and shoulders.

Usually missing from a physical examination by a mainstream physician is the physical manipulation of the spine and back area itself. Performed by knowledgeable and practiced hands, the touching of the muscles and bones of your back can provide a great deal of information about where tension and stress are being held and/or injury has taken place. One of the many benefits of more natural, holistic approaches to the prevention and treatment of back pain is the physical, personal contact between healer and patient.

DIAGNOSTIC PROCEDURES

After the history and the physical examination are completed, your physician may want to perform diagnostic tests, usually to confirm the suspected diagnosis and to rule out some serious, but far less likely, causes of back pain. Among the tests included are these:

Lab Tests. Your doctor may suggest performing urine and blood testing designed to rule out the possibility that the pain is being caused by an infection or other serious ailment, especially if your pain is accompanied by fever.

X-ray. The most common test performed for back pain is also, unfortunately, generally the most useless. Because x-rays show only bone, any muscle or other soft-tissue problems—the cause of at least 70 percent of all back pain—will not be evident.

Depending on what your medical history and x-ray and lab screening indicate, you may be considered a candidate for further testing using more sophisticated diagnostic tools. Such testing is usually suggested only when surgery is indicated. It is important to emphasize that even if these tests show a spinal abnormality, this may not be the cause of your back pain. A second opinion, perhaps by a holistic practitioner in one of the disciplines described in this book, should be obtained before decisions about surgery or other radical treatment are made.

CT Scan. Computed tomography—the CT scan—is a process that works by "photographing" the spine in several cross sections, thereby viewing the interior tissues as well as those on the surface. In general, CT scans should only be used to look for tumors or fractures of the vertebrae themselves. The test is not painful, only time-consuming. The average lumbar spine CT scan takes about 20 to 40 minutes, during which an individual lies flat on an x-ray table. However, CT scans may be prohibitively expensive, ranging in cost from $700 to $800, and not available in all areas.

MRI. Technologically speaking, the MRI (magnetic resonance imaging) is another step up from the CT scan. This test is capable of depicting the spine in many planes—front, back, side, and down through the spinal canal. It is capable of diagnosing everything from herniated discs to compressed nerves and spinal tumors. The procedure from the patient's perspective is about the same as for a CT scan: lying flat and still on a table for about 30 to 60 minutes. An MRI may be indicated if your physician feels your problem is particularly puzzling or intractable but, again, is unnecessary in the majority of cases.

Bone Scan. This test, which uses radiolabeled molecules to see if some areas of bone are growing faster than others, is generally used only to determine the spread of cancer. It is rarely used at all today, having been largely replaced by the CT scan.

EMG Study. Electromyography studies the electrical activity of muscles both at rest and during contraction. In this procedure, electrodes are placed on the skin and a weak electrical current is passed through them while the activity of nerves and muscles is recorded. An EMG study is used to diagnose diseases such as muscular dystrophy and injuries such as nerve entrapment.

Once your history, lab tests, and related diagnostic procedures are evaluated, your doctor will work with you to develop a treatment plan.

Outlining the Solutions

For Tim and Karen, and the millions of other Americans who will suffer from back pain this year, the plain truth of the matter is that modern mainstream medicine has little to offer in the way of a permanent cure for their condition. Standard mainstream medicine offers two main therapeutic options to the chronic back pain sufferer: drug therapy to relax muscles and relieve pain, and surgery to correct perceived injuries or malformation of the bones, discs, and joints of the spine.

Drug Therapy. There are several drugs commonly prescribed to control—never to "cure"—back pain. Some are mild and some are quite potent. Like all drugs, each has its risks for side effects that should be weighed against the potential benefit.

There are several types of drugs that might be prescribed for back pain. Analgesics (painkillers like the over-the-counter Tylenol and the prescription drug Darvon) are commonly used, as are nonsteroidal antiinflammatory drugs (like aspirin, ibuprofen, and stronger prescription medications such as Motrin, Feldene, Naprosyn, and indomethacin). Other drug options are muscle relaxants such as Flexeril and Robaxin; antianxiety drugs such as Valium and Xanax, which also act as smooth-muscle relaxants; and narcotics such as codeine and Percodan. Elavil, an antidepressant, may be given in small doses to help relieve chronic pain.

Except for the milder analgesics and antiinflammatory drugs, all of these medications are potentially addictive drugs with serious short- and long-term side effects. One can even become overly dependent on aspirin and ibuprofen to mask the pain, without ever getting closer to finding a permanent solution to the underlying problems. In addition, aspirin and other NSAIDs may irritate the stomach, eventually causing bleeding and/or gastritis.

Without doubt, a muscle relaxer can save you if you are felled by an excruciating muscle spasm. Aspirin or ibuprofen can relieve the inflammation and achiness that often follow a minor injury or strain. But if you find yourself taking medication on a daily basis, and before you decide to take stronger narcotics or antianxiety drugs, try to find out what physical and/or emotional problems are causing your back pain and look toward solving them with one or more of the natural and holistic models outlined in this book.

Surgery. More than 200,000 Americans undergo surgery to treat their back pain every year, but according to several different studies, only about 25 percent report feeling a dramatic improvement in their conditions following the procedure. In fact, according to Norman Shealy, M.D., former president of the American Holistic Medical Association and prominent neurosurgeon, fewer than 1 percent of all back pain sufferers have disc problems requiring surgery.

The most common surgical procedures for back pain are the laminectomy, in which a disc believed to be damaged is removed along with part of the corresponding vertebra, and the discectomy, in which the part of the disc that impinges on a nerve is cut away. Surgeons have been performing these procedures for several decades, and apart from the general risks of anesthesia, they are safe for most people. In addition, newer microsurgery techniques are even less invasive in removing the damaged portions of discs. However, in general, these procedures all require hospitalization and a postoperative rehabilitation period and thus should not be undertaken lightly, especially when the benefits of surgery are far from clear in most cases.

The truth of the matter is that about 90 percent of all cases of back pain will resolve themselves—without any treatment at all—within two weeks. That said, it is likely that in a vast majority of these same cases, back pain will recur, and recur often, unless the underlying problems are resolved. In Chapter 2, you learned some of the day-to-day mistakes we make in posture, simple movements, exercise—even in rest—that place undue stress and strain on the back. We've also discussed how important our emotional and spiritual lives are to the state of our general health. How we think and feel about ourselves and our place in the universe may have a great deal of impact on the condition of our spinal cord and back muscles.

In short, most cases of back pain result from a combination of physical and emotional factors that go far beyond what can be shown on an x-ray or, in the vast majority of cases, what can be resolved by surgery. If you are one of the millions of Americans who will suffer from either an acute or a chronic back pain problem this year, it is important for you to gain a deeper understanding not only of the anatomy and physiology of your musculoskeletal system, but of your general lifestyle and emotional state as well. The chapters that follow will help you explore some of these issues as they explain the way alternative therapies can be used to prevent and treat one of the most common and debilitating conditions of modern times: back pain.

"*It is no*

rest to be idle."

Paul Peel

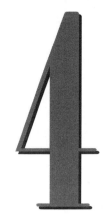

Exercise: The Path to a Healthy Back

$\mathcal{S}$ome forty years ago, long before the current (and largely artificial) fitness fad began, an interesting new term was coined by renowned back ailment expert, Hans Kraus, M.D. In Dr. Kraus's opinion, the American people were suffering from an epidemic of what he called "hypokinetic diseases": conditions largely caused by the lack of exercise. Under this umbrella stood such chronic and potentially fatal ailments as heart disease, stroke, high blood pressure, and certain cancers. By failing to move our bodies, open our lungs, and work our muscles, Dr. Kraus postulated, we were dooming ourselves to a host of often preventable diseases.

Back pain, the second most common complaint among adults in this country then and now, represented to Dr. Kraus a classic example of a hypokinetic disease, one that results from having lax, weak muscles that can no longer do the job they were designed to do—keeping our bodies in balance and harmony in motion and at rest. A man ahead of his time, Kraus also warned against the increasing level of stress to which the modern population was being subjected, and the damaging impact that it had on the health of our musculoskeletal system.

Unfortunately, Dr. Kraus's messages fell upon apparently deaf ears. A study performed by the National Center for Health Statistics and published in the July, 1994, issue of the *Journal of the American Medical Association* proved that nearly one third of all Americans remain obese, that is, 20 percent or more above a healthy weight. Although fitness tests to measure cardiovascular endurance and muscular strength were not performed, fewer than 50 percent of those surveyed did any kind of exercise on a regular basis. The result of these two factors—overweight and lack of exercise—is that cardiovascular disease remains the nation's number one killer and back pain a significant problem for millions of American men and women.

Before we rush to judgment and admonish ourselves for being lazy and unmotivated, it is important that we recognize the powerful forces aligned against us on the road to health and fitness. Most of us live in a world driven by very mixed media messages about weight,

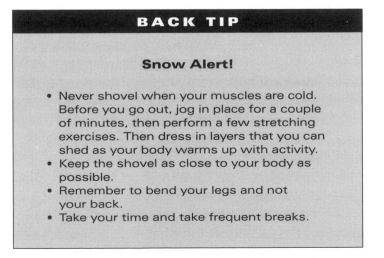

BACK TIP

Snow Alert!

- Never shovel when your muscles are cold. Before you go out, jog in place for a couple of minutes, then perform a few stretching exercises. Then dress in layers that you can shed as your body warms up with activity.
- Keep the shovel as close to your body as possible.
- Remember to bend your legs and not your back.
- Take your time and take frequent breaks.

body image, and lifestyle. We see rail-thin models advertising fat-laden potato chips and athletes peddling beer. We are prodded to buy time- and physical-energy saving devices like power-driven lawnmowers, snow shovels, and dishwashers. The television set beckons to us con-stantly, urging us to relinquish the physical in favor of the passive, and too many of us give in and spend from six to eight hours every day in front of the tube.

Breaking out of this cycle of inactivity and chronic disease takes time, energy, and commitment. It also requires us to peel back the lay-ers of misinformation, apathy, and frustration about health and fitness that may have built up over the years. Eating a proper diet *will* make you feel better and can be every bit as tasty and enticing as the foods you see advertised. Reading a book or learning a new hobby is *more* relaxing than passively watching television hour after hour.

And as for exercise, it is a positive life-enhancing habit that pro-motes physical and emotional health and well-being—not a painful, tedious grind. Properly performed on a regular basis, exercise allows you to connect with your physical body in an intimate way. You'll be able to feel your muscles grow stronger, your heart beat more rigor-ously, and your nervous system throw off the built-up tension and stress of the day. Balance will be restored, balance within your body and balance between you and the rest of the physical world. With every hour we spend in the artificial environment of television, fax machines, and stuffy offices, the farther we get from nature and the true role we are meant to play within it.

EXERCISE AND YOUR HEALTH

In the 1985 edition of the Signet/Mosby *Medical Encyclopedia,* exercise is defined as "any action or skill that exerts the muscles and is performed in order to condition the body, improve health, or maintain fitness." Specifically, exercise helps the body to perform its vital func-tions in the following ways:

Exercise increases the efficiency of the heart and blood vessels. The cardiovascular system has as its primary function the delivery of oxygen, an element essential to life, to every cell in the body. With regular aerobic exercise (exercise that requires oxygen for energy), the heart and vessels are able to pump more blood and thus deliver more oxygen and other nutrients to all the muscles of the body, including those of the back, with greater efficiency. Furthermore, exercise helps keep blood pressure and blood cholesterol at normal levels, thus reducing the risk of heart disease and high blood pressure—which remain the nation's number one health problem.

Exercise promotes deep breathing. Oxygen is more vital to our health and well-being than perhaps any other single nutrient or activity. Nevertheless, few of us fully appreciate how important it is to breathe deeply in order to fully expand the lungs and bathe the cells in oxygen-rich blood. During vigorous and sustained exercise, an adult breathes about twice as fast and much more deeply than he or she does at rest, increasing intake from 10 to approximately 20 gallons of air per minute.

In addition, according to many Eastern philosophies, the breath is more than a way to physically sustain the life force of cells. It is also the vehicle of the original cosmic energy that has brought everything else into being. According to these traditions, how much and how often we take in oxygen controls how energy deeply affects the health of the body and mind.

Exercise stretches and strengthens muscles. Of primary importance to anyone interested in preventing or alleviating back pain is the development of strong, flexible muscles. Well-conditioned muscles help you perform daily tasks of all sorts (including merely sitting down) with more efficiency and less strain. You are more likely to maintain proper posture if your spine, hips, and shoulders are supported by a strong musculature. A trim waist and flat stomach reduce pressure on the lower back. Good flexibility protects the muscles against pulls and tears; short, tight muscles are likely to become injured during even moderate activity.

Exercise maintains the body's proper metabolism. More Americans than ever before are obese, a problem that no doubt contributes to most cases of back pain. With exercise, however, maintaining a healthy weight comes almost naturally, especially if paired with a relatively sensible low-fat, high-fiber diet. First, through regular aerobic exercise, your body learns to burn stored fat more efficiently to use as fuel to meet its increased energy needs. Second, muscle is more metabolically active than fat. The body must burn more calories to feed and nourish muscle tissue than it would to maintain fat. Therefore, the more muscle you have, the more calories you'll burn every day.

Exercise allows the body and the mind to relax. According to Hans Kraus, M.D.—and more and more mainstream and alternative practitioners every day—stress plays a significant role in the development of many cases of back pain. With tension, the muscles of your shoulders, neck, and lower back tighten. If they fail to relax, they lose their suppleness and, over time, they become permanently shortened and actually lose their ability to release tension. Only by working those muscles will the stress of the day (or the year!) ever be released.

Another benefit of exercise is that certain body chemicals called endorphins, known to dull pain and invoke mild euphoria, are released whenever the body feels pain, including during vigorous exercise when the muscles begin to tire and "burn." Produced in the spinal cord and the brain, endorphins serve as a perfect example of the body's power to return itself to a state of balance and may be the reason that exercise appears to reduce anxiety and stress in those who undertake it on a regular basis.

For all of these reasons—for your general health and the health of your back—you should begin to make exercise a part of your daily life. In this chapter, we briefly cover the three categories of exercise necessary to achieve overall fitness, which will help you maintain a healthy back: stretching, strengthening, and aerobics.

If you suffer from chronic or acute back pain, it is important for you to receive proper guidance from your physician, alternative practitioner, and/or a physical therapist/trainer before you begin to exercise. As careful as we might be to describe exercises properly, nothing beats having someone watch the way your unique muscles work while you exercise, steer you to the exercises that will provide you with the most benefit, then make sure you are performing them efficiently and in good form.

An Exercise Program for a Healthy Back

Generally speaking, a healthy exercise program consists of three basic components: stretching, strengthening, and aerobic conditioning. Some of the most effective exercises for helping prevent and alleviate back pain are provided below.

STRETCHING

Many Americans neglect flexibility, even those who consider themselves to be in top physical condition. Part of the reason may lie in the noncompetitive nature of stretching. Unlike aerobics and weight training, there are no times or weight limits to beat. Instead, stretching the muscles slowly and steadily to their limit and slightly beyond requires an intensely personal effort, one that will bring you closer to truly understanding the unique structure of your own body. Stretching increases the range of motion of a joint as well as increases the blood supply to the muscle, thereby reducing the chance of injury or strain.

Stretching should always be preceded by a brief warm-up, such as light jogging in place, a few minutes on a stationary bicycle, or a brisk five-minute walk, to increase blood flow to the muscles. When you stretch, you should never jerk or bounce. Instead, the movements should be slow and fluid, and each position should be held for 10 or 12 seconds at a time. Breathe deeply as you stretch to allow your muscles to enjoy the full benefit of the stretch, as well as to more deeply relax and repair themselves when the position is released. Yoga exercises, which stretch muscles slowly and steadily while bathing the cells in oxygen through deep breathing, are particularly effective in promoting flexibility and increased circulation. (See Chapter 10 for more information.)

Among the stretching exercises designed to increase the flexibility of your back are the following:

Pelvic Tilt. Lie on your back, with knees bent. Hold in your stomach and tighten your buttock muscles. Keeping both feet and your lower back flat on the floor, lift your hips up off the floor and hold the position for 10 seconds. Release slowly. Repeat.

Lower Back Stretch. Lie on your back, legs straight in front of you. Grasp behind one knee and, bending that leg while keeping the other leg straight, pull it toward your chin. Hold that position for 10 seconds. Repeat.

Lower Back Curl. Lying flat on your back, lift one leg in the air to a 45-degree angle, then slowly lower it over the opposite side of your body (probably at about hip level). Keep your lower back and your hips anchored to the floor. Hold the stretch for 10 seconds or so, then repeat on the other side.

Cat Stretch. Assume a crawling position with your hands and your knees on the floor. Slowly and gently arch your back, much like a cat does upon awakening from one of its many naps. As you do so, drop your head down, bringing your chin close to your chest. Hold the stretch for about 10 seconds, then slowly lift your head and flatten your back. From this position, pull your shoulders back and lift your hips, so that you are in a semi-swayback position; hold for 10 seconds. Then repeat both postures to fully stretch all the muscles of your back.

Leg Lifts. Lie on your back with your legs straight out in front of you. Slowly lift one leg straight into the air, which will gently stretch your lower back. Hold this pose for 10 seconds, then slowly lower your leg. Repeat with other leg.

Thigh Stretches. Lie on your back with your knees bent, and your feet on the floor. Place your hands on the insides of your thighs and gently drop your knees outward to stretch your groin and thigh muscles.

In addition to these specific back stretches, there are some that work other parts of the body. Since overall fitness and flexibility should be your ultimate goal, we suggest that you include these stretches as part of your daily routine:

Shoulders/Upper Back. Raise your right arm and reach down your back as far as you can. At the same time, place your left arm behind your back and try to reach the fingers of your right hand. Sustain this stretch for 5 to 10 seconds. Repeat with arms reversed.

Chest/Arms. Stand sideways and at arm's length from a wall. Reach out and slightly behind you and place one palm on the wall. Keeping your hand in place, turn your body away slightly. Hold the stretch for 5 to 10 seconds. Face the other direction and repeat with the other arm.

Calves. Lean forward on the balls of your feet, heels lifted, and bounce, very gently, 20 times. Then, at slightly less than arm's length and with heels on the floor, lean toward a wall, supporting your weight on both hands. Keep your legs straight and heels on the ground. Hold the stretch for 10 seconds.

Hamstrings. Place one foot about 12 inches in front of the other. Raise the toes of the leading foot in the air. Keeping both knees slightly bent, lean your torso forward as if you were taking a bow. Feel the stretch, for about 10 seconds, in the back and front of your thigh. Reverse the position.

STRENGTHENING

For the individual with back pain, strengthening the muscles that support the spine is essential, particularly the abdominal muscles, the hip flexors, and the muscles of the shoulders and chest. In addition, overall muscle strength and endurance are critical to your general health and fitness. Every muscle in your body plays a role in keeping you standing tall, moving smoothly, and sitting properly.

You achieve muscle strength and endurance by applying resistance to normal body motion. The resistance, or load, causes muscles to contract with an increased tension. You can add resistance in two ways: through the weight of your own body in a series of exercises called calisthenics (sit-ups, push-ups, etc.) and by using adjustable weights. Because the techniques of calisthenics and weight training are very precise and, if not performed properly, can lead to injury, we suggest that you visit a local gym or YMCA to receive firsthand instruction before you begin a program on your own.

A weight-training routine should involve about 30 minutes of slow but constant stress on different muscles of the body using your own body weight (calisthenics), free weights, or strength-training equipment (such as Nautilus). Your exact exercise routine should be formulated with an exercise specialist in a gym, but generally speaking it should consist of about a dozen exercises: six for the upper body and six for the lower. Of most importance to the average person with back pain are exercises designed to firm and tone the abdomen, shoulders, buttocks, and hip flexors.

For most people with back pain, the abdominal curl is an especially helpful exercise, which is why we've included it here. Also known as the sit-up, the abdominal curl is designed to help strengthen your abdominal muscles, which in turn, help keep your back strong and supple. Your abdominals wrap three quarters of the way around your lower back, offering your spine a great deal of support if they themselves are in shape.

Proper form is crucial in performing the abdominal curl. In fact, you will be doing your back more harm than good if you fail to follow with care the directions outlined below. If you experience back pain during or following this exercise, consider obtaining advice about your form from a trained exercise professional at your local YMCA or gym.

Please note: Anaerobic exercises, which include calisthenics and weight training (with free weights or with Nautilus), are not usually recommended for people with high blood pressure or advanced cardiovascular disease of any type. Such exercises may cause temporary but marked rises in blood pressure. If you suffer from high blood pressure and/or heart disease, or if you are over 40 and are new to weight training, talk to your physician and/or alternative practitioner before doing these kinds of exercises.

Abdominal Curl. Lie on your back with your knees bent, pressing your lower back into the floor. Tuck your chin close to your chest and place your hands between your thighs or across your chest. Tighten your abdominal muscles, allowing them to lift your upper body until your shoulders are off the floor. Hold this position for 3 seconds, then slowly return to the original position. Repeat this exercise 10–20 times.

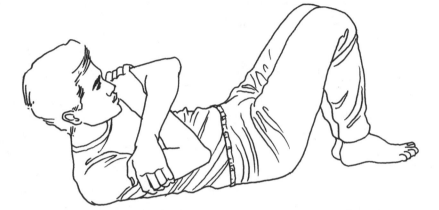

Proper Sit-Up

*Strengthening your abdominal muscles is an important
way to provide support for the spine and back. To perform a correct
sit-up, lie on your back with your feet flat on the floor and your
knees raised. Cross your arms on your chest. Then tuck your chin close
to your chest and gently lift your shoulders off the floor. As
you tighten your abdominal muscles, try to reach your elbows to
your knees. The movement will be small—you'll move
just 1 or 2 inches. Try to do 20 repetitions, rest for a minute,
then repeat the exercise.*

AEROBIC EXERCISE

Aerobic exercises are those activities that promote cardiovascular fitness by enhancing the body's ability to deliver large amounts of oxygen to working muscles. Aerobic exercises generally involve working large muscle groups (such as leg muscles) for a sustained length of time, generally more than 20 minutes at a steady, moderate pace. In addition to furthering cardiovascular health, aerobic exercise increases your body's ability to burn fat more efficiently for fuel, a definite boon for people trying to lose excess weight and reduce the burden of extra weight on the muscles of the back.

There are literally dozens of activities that can provide aerobic benefits if performed over a sustained period of time—at least 20 to 30 minutes—including walking, aerobic dance, cross-country skiing, cycling, swimming, ice skating, running, and jogging. However, some activities tend to involve a bit more risk to the muscles of the back than others and should be undertaken only with extreme care.

If you enjoy a sport or exercise that you find to be painful or if you are fearful that pain might occur if you attempt it, talk to a trained physical therapist or fitness trainer. He or she may be able to help you modify the activity or work with you until you feel more comfortable. Remember, a prime benefit of exercise is the sense of release and relaxation it offers. You should enjoy this time of your day, not be held prisoner by either the activity itself or any anxiety you may feel about performing it.

Here is a list of the most common aerobic activities along with a description of how they might affect a person who suffers with chronic back problems:

Low-Risk Activities

- *Walking:* Perhaps the best overall exercise for those with and without back problems, walking puts less strain on the spine than jogging, running, or surprisingly even sitting still for long periods of time.
- *Swimming:* Because water supports the spine, swimming tends to relieve the pressure on it. The backstroke and sidestroke are

best for the back. The butterfly and breaststroke, on the other hand, which cause you to arch the back, are not recommended for those with back pain.

- *Bicycling:* Provided you maintain an upright posture, stationary or outdoor cycling is an excellent aerobic exercise that can be done without much risk to your back. Make sure the handle bars and seats are properly adjusted so that you don't have to hunch over when you pedal. Also be sure to straighten your legs completely when pedaling so that you stretch your hamstring muscles in the back of your thighs.

Higher-risk Activities

- *Jogging/Running:* The jury is still out on whether jogging and running are bad or good for your back, but it does appear that these activities place a great deal of stress on other bones and joints of the body, particularly the ankles and the knees. And if any part of your body becomes injured or misaligned, your back can ultimately suffer as well. For that reason, jogging and running should be undertaken only with caution—and make sure you warm up before you stretch, and stretch before you run.
- *Golf:* One survey found that 25 percent of all golf pros suffer from chronic low back injuries. Because golf requires much stooping and bending (to tee the ball, retrieve the ball from the cup, prolonged putting practice) as well as twisting and turning, this activity can exacerbate back problems. If you have a weak back, such movements can put enormous extra pressure on the spine and lower back. Walking the golf course, may provide some aerobic benefit, but carrying your heavy golf bag yourself may cause you to injure your back.
- *Tennis and Other Racquet Sports:* Like golf, tennis, racquetball, and squash require a great deal of twisting and arching of the back, as well as plenty of sudden starts and stops. On the other hand, these sports are fun, can provide aerobic benefits if performed at a sufficient level of play, and certainly work important muscles like the shoulders, chest, and hip flexors. If you

would like to play tennis or another racquet sport, start slowly and be sure to stop if you feel any pain.

- *Football, Basketball, Baseball:* In addition to the bending, lifting, and stop-and-start aspects of play, these sports often involve sliding, falling, jumping, and contact with other players. If you have a weak back, it would be best to avoid these activities until you feel stronger.

General Guidelines

In the best of all possible worlds, every one of us would get out of bed bright and early, take a few deep breaths, run in place for a few minutes, gently stretch our muscles, then take a brisk walk, a short jog, or play a set of tennis. But for most of us, that scenario is not a reality. Instead, we must work exercise into our lives, slowly but surely making it part of our weekly, if not our daily, routine.

If possible, and especially if you are currently suffering from back pain, try every day to do the stretches outlined in this chapter. Including the warm-up, this routine should take no more than 10 minutes.

As for strengthening your muscles and increasing your aerobic capabilities, you should aim for exercising about three to five days per week for about 30 minutes at a time. Don't get discouraged if you are not able to meet that schedule at first. Every time you move your body, you're doing something positive for your health, even if it's just for 10 extra minutes a day. On the other hand, to really experience a difference in the way you feel about your body and your health, you'll need to make exercise a regular part of your life.

Here are a few tips to get you started on the road to fitness:

Check with Your Doctor or Practitioner. Your first step in starting an exercise program is to consult with your physician and/or alternative practitioner, especially if you're overweight, over 40, or have any other risk factors for cardiovascular disease. Your health practitioner may recommend that you take a stress test, which mea-

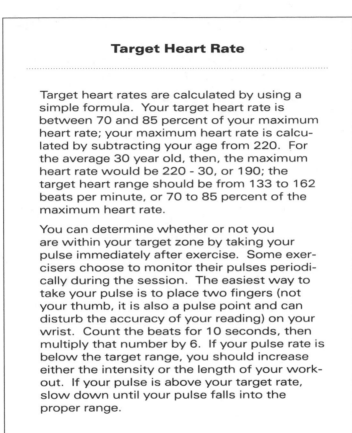

Target Heart Rate

Target heart rates are calculated by using a simple formula. Your target heart rate is between 70 and 85 percent of your maximum heart rate; your maximum heart rate is calculated by subtracting your age from 220. For the average 30 year old, then, the maximum heart rate would be 220 - 30, or 190; the target heart range should be from 133 to 162 beats per minute, or 70 to 85 percent of the maximum heart rate.

You can determine whether or not you are within your target zone by taking your pulse immediately after exercise. Some exercisers choose to monitor their pulses periodically during the session. The easiest way to take your pulse is to place two fingers (not your thumb, it is also a pulse point and can disturb the accuracy of your reading) on your wrist. Count the beats for 10 seconds, then multiply that number by 6. If your pulse rate is below the target range, you should increase either the intensity or the length of your workout. If your pulse is above your target rate, slow down until your pulse falls into the proper range.

sures how your heart and blood vessels are functioning. Both the length of time you are able to exercise and the intensity of activity you are able to endure without becoming exhausted will help your doctor determine a safe exercise routine for you.

Start Slow. A study published in the *Journal of the American Medical Association* in November, 1989, showed that moderate exercise—defined as 30 minutes a day of light activity such as walking and gardening—is almost as beneficial to one's health as higher levels of exercise, such as high-impact aerobics and jogging. Moreover, moderate exercise is far safer than high-intensity activities.

Choose Activities You Enjoy. Perhaps the most important element in the design of your exercise program is choosing activities you will enjoy over the long haul. Think of it this way: If you exercise three times a week for 30 minutes a session, you'll have stair-stepped, jogged, or rowed for about 78 hours—the equivalent of two solid workweeks—at the end of a year.

Wear Proper Footwear. Although there is no need for you to spend lots of money on fancy walking shoes or aerobic sneakers, you should choose a shoe that has a rigid arch and some cushioning on the heel and ball of the foot. Such support will help keep your body properly aligned as you walk or perform any other aerobic activity.

Set Realistic Goals. If you've been sedentary for a number of months or years, deciding to train for next month's marathon by running 10 miles every morning would be counterproductive and even dangerous to your health, especially if you suffer from back pain. After failing to meet the unrealistic goal, or straining your back trying to do so, you'd become frustrated and probably decide not to exercise at all. Instead, set goals you know you can meet, or perhaps ones just barely out of reach. Achieving them will give you a sense of pride and self-confidence sure to keep you motivated.

Vary Your Routine. Plan two or three different workout routines in addition to stretching every day. Bicycle one day, walk the next, try a new sport (once you feel your back is in good shape) the next. This will cut back on the chances you'll get bored with your exercise program, a prime reason that many of us end up giving up our resolve and going back to being couch potatoes.

Find a Support Group. For most of us, there comes a time when our motivation sags and we lose interest in exercising on a regular basis. When this happens—preferably *before* this happens—enlist a friend or loved one to join you in your fitness quest.

Regular exercise has another special benefit to those who suffer from chronic back pain: It serves to release the tension and stress that usually take their largest toll on the muscles of the neck, shoulders, and lower back. In Chapter 5, we'll describe other techniques for relieving emotional pressures.

"If you fail
to plan, you
plan to fail."

Old saying

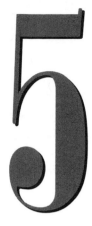

Relaxing
Out of the Pain

abe Wilson, *a computer programmer with a high-tech, high-stress job, cannot remember a time when he didn't suffer with back pain. The pain tended to build during the day as he sat at his computer terminal, sometimes bothering him so much that he needed to stop his car on the way home and get out to stretch his back. Finally, he decided to visit a doctor for an evaluation.*

On the advice of the physician, Gabe submitted to an MRI of the lower back, a sophisticated x-ray that showed no disc problems or other abnormalities. His doctor then prescribed antiinflammatory medication for Gabe to take on a regular basis and suggested a course of exercises intended to stretch and strengthen his back muscles.

A television show about biofeedback and its usefulness in controlling chronic pain prompted Gabe to visit a specialist at a local stress reduction clinic. The biofeedback practitioner had a technique that surprised Gabe: Not only did she examine him and look at his x-rays, but she spent a great deal of time asking questions about every detail of his life, focusing on what his daily routine was like, what tended to give him the most stress during the day and how he usually coped with it, and even his general emotional and spiritual state.

She then demonstrated the biofeedback equipment. First she placed small patches, called electrodes, on the skin above the tight muscles in his back and then connected the electrodes to a computer screen. The electrodes measured the amount of tension in the muscles and translated that amount into a graph on the computer screen. The biofeedback specialist then led Gabe through some guided imagery meant to relax him. He imagined himself floating on clear, warm water, and as he did so, he felt the tension drain away from his body. As his muscles relaxed, the electrodes transmitted that information to the computer and he could see changes on the graph.

The next step in the process involved attaching temperature sensors to Gabe's fingers. After exercising his fingers to warm them up, Gabe then cooled them down in a cup of cold water. The specialist explained that his fingers warmed up because blood flows to tissues more rapidly during exercise or during times of stress. Learning to warm the fingers as measured on the sensor was a good way to learn to control the part of the nervous system that responds to physical or emotional stress. By learning to relax this system, Gabe could release his feelings of stress, which in him included spasm of the back muscles.

The specialist gave Gabe several meditation exercises to perform at home, and asked him to come back the next week. Soon Gabe was able to clearly alter the graph by relaxing—both by lowering his finger temperature and by relaxing his muscles. The therapist gave Gabe a number of suggestions to help him reduce his stress at work and at home, including taking more short breaks away from his computer terminal, breathing deeply, eating properly, and more openly expressing his dissatisfaction instead of letting it build to become simmering anger, resentment, and muscle tension. She also suggested that he use a better office chair and drive with a cushion behind his lower back.

After a few sessions, Gabe realized that he was having less back pain on a daily basis. Even more exciting, he was beginning to be able to automatically relax and breathe deeply whenever he felt stressed or tense. His wife and co-workers all commented on how much more relaxed and calm Gabe seemed.

THE CYCLE OF PAIN

Gabe Wilson's case of chronic back pain stems from an all too common succession of events in the lives of modern Americans. Indeed, pain and anxiety are two separate feelings that often form one vicious cycle, one that traps and torments many people who suffer from back pain. Stress and anxiety might start the cycle, causing neck, shoulder, and lower back muscles to tighten and eventually to ache. Over time, these muscles may become shortened and thus more vulnerable to strains and tears. As the pain continues, the person who suffers from it begins to worry about what's causing the discomfort and about doing anything that might make it worse. Worry turns to chronic anxiety, adding to the original problem and keeping the cycle in motion. In other cases, a physical injury occurs first, followed by stress and anxiety. In either instance, the pain remains chronic and intractable unless the individual learns to break the cycle.

With biofeedback, Gabe Wilson found a way out of his cycle of pain and frustration. Others have found that hypnotherapy, guided imagery, and/or meditation help them return to a state of balance and health. In this chapter, we'll discuss these and other approaches and how they are used to treat back pain. First, however, we need to take a look at the physiology of pain and its relationship to stress.

The Path of Pain

There are two basic types of pain: acute and chronic. Acute pain is a warning system, a message from the body that something is wrong and needs attention. When your back muscles go into spasm, for instance, the ensuing pain protects your muscles from further damage by preventing you from being able to move. Acute pain eventually resolves itself when the danger has passed and the trigger—the cause of the spasm—has been released.

Chronic pain, on the other hand, continues for long periods of time and, apparently, serves no useful physiological function. Your body somehow becomes "stuck" within the pain, caught in the cycle of frustration, pain, and exhaustion outlined above. Chronic pain is no less real or serious than acute pain. In fact, chronic pain may point to deeper, more intractable physical and emotional problems, requiring more, not less, attention and commitment to treat.

Acute or chronic, pain is a very individual and personal matter. No two people experience pain or find relief from it in exactly the same way. Although a fracture of the wrist bone or a cavity in a molar appears to do the same amount of damage in any two individuals, the way pain is perceived by each of them may be completely different: One might be in agony while the other complains of only minor discomfort.

The word "perception" is an important one when it comes to a discussion of pain and our response to it. That's because the pathway

BACK TIP

Take Frequent
Meditation Breaks

Relaxing away the stresses of the day needn't be an elaborate affair. Whenever you feel particularly tense, just close your eyes and visualize a calm, pleasant scene, like floating in cool, fresh water or sitting beneath twinkling stars on a clear evening. For a few minutes, let your body live in that scene and soon you'll feel your muscles relax and your spirit begin to soar.

from stimulation (injury) to response (ouch!) is not a straight one. When you burn your finger on a stove, for instance, the sensation of pain travels along a series of nerve fibers from your finger to the brain. There are many ways that the pain message may be altered or even canceled along the route.

Perhaps the most important way that the body protects itself against pain is by producing substances called endorphins. (Endorphins are chemicals produced in the brain, spinal cord, and elsewhere in the body in response to the perception of pain.) Once released, these chemicals are able to attach to certain receptors in the brain and throughout the body, thereby dulling the perception of pain. In fact, man-made opiates such as morphine and heroin have a chemical structure similar to that of endorphins, which accounts for their painkilling capacities.

The brain produces endorphins under a number of different conditions, including exercise, meditation, and the stimulation of acupuncture points. In addition, certain emotions and emotional responses appear to either trigger or hinder the release of endorphins. Some studies indicate that depression, a common side effect of chronic pain, for instance, decreases endorphin production, while laughter increases production. Self-esteem is an extremely important, and often overlooked, aspect of health. Those who feel that they are destined to fail (and thus have no control over their lives) or are unworthy of the success they do achieve, tend to feel stress and pain more acutely than others with more confidence in themselves and their ability to alter their environment. Indeed, our emotional lives have a direct bearing on all aspects of our physical health, including the state of the muscles, tendons, and nerves in our backs.

Stress and Back Pain

Once your brain perceives pain of any kind, several different hormones are produced that stimulate a number of physical and emotional reactions. When you are frightened by the pain and/or what caused it, for instance, your palms may begin to sweat, your heart rate and blood pressure to rise, and your muscles to contract. Known as the "fight-or-flight" response, this is an automatic reaction meant to keep us safe from any situation that we perceive as dangerous. It prepares us either to stay and fight the "enemy" (in this case whatever triggered the pain), or to flee. When this response is triggered over and over again by chronic pain, the end result may be more harmful than protective, however. It is, in fact, another form of stress that can weigh heavily on our minds and bodies.

One branch of the nervous system, called the autonomic nervous system, is particularly important in the fight-or-flight stress response. The autonomic nervous system regulates bodily functions like the heartbeat, intestinal movements, muscular contraction, and other activities of the internal organs. It is divided into two parts that work to balance these activities: The sympathetic nervous system speeds up heart rate, raises blood pressure, and tenses muscles during times of physical or emotional stress, while the parasympathetic nervous system works to slow these processes down when the body perceives that the stress has passed.

Indeed, the two parts of the autonomic system represent a perfect example of the balance we know of as health. In Chinese medicine, the sympathetic nervous system is the "yang" and the parasympathetic system is the "yin" of the body and its responses. Bringing your body into harmony during and after stressful periods by triggering your parasympathetic nervous system is as important to your health as is reacting immediately, through the sympathetic nervous system, to the perceived threats known as stressors.

Two of the most powerful stress-related hormones are called nor-epinephrine and epinephrine. These hormones stimulate the sympathetic nervous system to raise blood pressure and heart rate, to make you breathe in more oxygen, and to cause your muscles to tense up. If you remain under constant pain, your back muscles may become chronically and abnormally contracted and thus achy and subject to spasm.

At the same time, the more stress and pain you feel, the more likely it is that you will engage in high-risk behaviors, such as smoking and drinking too much, overeating, and exercising too little. Although you may feel that these habits help to relax you, they are, in fact, increasing the stress on your body and your back by forcing you to cope with the ill effects of these substances and behaviors.

The good news, however, is that within our bodies we have powerful weapons that can fight against chronic pain and stress. In short, we are naturally able to both boost our production of the natural painkillers called endorphins and, often at the same time, reduce the amount of debilitating, pain-producing "fight-or-flight" responses.

Controlling Pain through Stress Reduction

Although you may be under the impression that what you need to alleviate your back pain are drugs or surgery or exercise, it is unlikely that any of these methods will ultimately solve your problem if you remain under high levels of emotional and physical stress. At the same time that you undergo other treatment for your pain, you may want to examine some of the stress-related factors that may well be causing, or at least contributing to, your condition.

Is your job putting strain on your health? Your relationships? Your lack of physical activity? Do you live in a hostile environment, either physically or emotionally? If you can answer yes to any of these questions, you might want to consider ways to change your life in order to eliminate or at least alleviate these problems. Is it possible to change your job? Could you spare the time and money to receive family therapy to improve the way you relate to those close to you? Can you make stretching and strengthening exercises, such as those that were described in Chapter 4, a regular part of your life? Although making such fundamental changes may take a great deal of time and commitment on your part, the impact on your general state of fitness and health is likely to be enormous.

In the meantime, there are several more physical methods of stress reduction available to help you to bring your body back into balance quickly and efficiently during times of stress. In essence, you can learn to counteract the fight-or-flight response by activating your parasympathetic nervous system—your yin to counteract the overactive yang (sympathetic nervous system)—to attain a more peaceful and relaxed internal harmony. Biofeedback, hypnotherapy, guided imagery, meditation, and progressive relaxation are just a few of the many techniques known to help release physical and emotional tension. You should try a few different methods, each one for a week or two, before deciding which ones work best for you.

BIOFEEDBACK

Biofeedback is one of the most scientific methods for exploring and utilizing the mind-body connection. It is especially helpful for chronic pain sufferers like Gabe Wilson, whom you met at the beginning of this chapter, who can learn to use the power of their own mind to control and release their pain. The underlying premise behind biofeedback is that anyone can learn to modify his or her own vital functions—including heart rate, blood pressure, and muscle tension—by using his or her conscious mind. In other words, when properly trained, you can learn to relax the muscles of your back whenever you feel tightness and constriction beginning to take hold.

Biofeedback was developed when studies showed that animals could control bodily functions once thought to be completely automatic by being given a reward or a punishment. Physicians adapted those findings to design ways for humans to control unconscious functions through conscious thought. For Gabe Wilson and millions of others, this technique has spelled the end to years of frustration and aching muscles.

Although there are several biofeedback methods, they all have three things in common: (1) they measure a physiological function (such as muscle tension); (2) they convert this measurement to an understandable form (a computer-generated graph or chart like the kind that Gabe used, a blinking light, mercury levels in a thermometer, etc.); and (3) they feed back this information to the individual. As with all aspects of health care, it is important that you receive biofeedback therapy from a qualified practitioner. Generally speaking, that means someone with a firm grasp of both physiology and psychology who has been certified by the Biofeedback Certification Institute of America.

HYPNOTHERAPY

Hypnosis, or hypnotherapy, is a technique named for Hypnos, the Greek god of sleep. Since 1958, when the American Medical Association officially approved hypnotherapy as a tool for treating back pain, thousands of people have benefitted from its physically relaxing and emotionally releasing effects.

The goal of hypnotherapy is to bring your body and mind into a deeply relaxed state in order to make you more open to suggestion. Usually, a hypnotherapy session begins with the therapist asking you to close your eyes and think relaxing thoughts. With a soothing voice, the therapist guides you down a path of deeper and deeper relaxation by asking you to focus your attention on a word or an image. By doing so, the therapist hopes to quiet your conscious mind and to make the unconscious mind more accessible by blocking all outside thoughts and stimuli. Because the unconscious mind is less critical, suggestions have a better chance of taking effect than if you remained in a normal, alert state.

Once you are completely relaxed, the therapist may suggest that you experience your back pain in a different, more pleasant way, or picture the pain flowing out of your body in a stream. The therapist may also plant posthypnotic suggestions, ideas about your pain and pain relief that take effect after you awaken from the hypnotic state. These suggestions are designed to help you release the pain whenever it occurs. In the end, the ultimate goal is to give you a greater sense of control over your own pain.

When choosing a hypnotherapist, you should ask your doctor for suggestions as well as check with national training and licensing institutions, such as the American Institute of Hypnotherapy and the International Medical and Dental Hypnotherapy Association. (See *Natural Resources*, page 188, at the end of the book for more information.)

GUIDED IMAGERY

Related to hypnotherapy is another form of treatment for back pain that uses the power of the human mind as its basic weapon. The human imagination—that part of our hearts and minds that can picture and sense images and feelings—is one of the most potent health resources you have available to you. By utilizing the power of your mind, you can help evoke a physical response in your body in order to relax your muscles, stimulate your immune system, and reduce pain. In fact, guided imagery is now being used to treat any number of conditions in addition to back pain, including high blood pressure, gastrointestinal disorders, allergies, and premenstrual syndrome.

In addition to helping you relax your body, guided imagery also helps you access your emotions. By visualizing your back pain as a red and angry monster that you banish from your kingdom, for instance, you may learn to better understand how frustrated and sore the pain has made you feel, and how powerful and in control of your body you can be if given the chance to break the cycle.

Although it is possible to conduct your own guided imagery session, it is best when learning to have a trained professional, preferably someone who has experience with your particular type of back pain, develop a program for you and guide you through the steps until they become familiar. Talk to your doctor about finding a qualified therapist for you, or check in *Natural Resources*, page 188, for more information.

MEDITATION

Like biofeedback, hypnotherapy, and guided imagery, meditation is a mental exercise that affects body processes. The purpose of meditation for relaxation is to gain control over your thoughts so that you can choose what to focus upon and thus to let the stress flow out of your body. Meditation for relaxation requires no special training, and can be done at any time of day, and in any comfortable space. All it takes is about 15 minutes of uninterrupted quiet.

Meditation is effective both in reducing general stress and in helping to relax muscles made tense by anxiety or worry. When you meditate, you quiet the sympathetic nervous system, thereby reducing your heart rate and state of muscle contraction. In addition to its physical benefits, meditation can help you psychologically by allowing you to focus on the cause of your stress and to find ways to change the way you respond to the challenges you face. Researchers have found that meditation is related to greater self-actualization, more positive feelings after encountering a stressful situation, improvement in sleep behavior, and even an increased ability to quit smoking.

There are many good books on meditation available on the market that go into great detail about the proper sitting positions, what to expect, even what mental phrases to use. And there are schools of meditation that train both doctors and lay people in the intricacies of the meditative process. But the basic elements of meditation are very simple, and can be mastered by anyone willing to set aside a few minutes a day. An easy meditation exercise follows:

Basic Meditation Exercise

This is a simple meditation exercise that can help you relax and focus your attention away from the things that cause stress in your life. Start by sitting a few minutes—perhaps just 5 to 10—until the practice becomes comfortable to you. (If you are interested in learning more about meditation, see *Natural Resources*, page 188.)

1. Make sure you are wearing comfortable, loose, nonbinding clothing. Sweatpants or shorts and a T-shirt are ideal.
2. Find a quiet place where you will not be disturbed. Try not to sit any place where you might be easily distracted, such as in front of a window.
3. Sit on the floor in a comfortable position. If you can't sit on the floor comfortably, sit in a straight-backed chair.
4. Allow your hands to rest on your legs.
5. Lower your gaze so that your eyes are almost, but not quite, closed.
6. Take a deep breath and let it out slowly.

7. The easiest way to begin meditation is to count your breaths. Inhale, count one. Exhale, count two. Inhale, count three. Exhale, count four. Do this to ten, and then start again with one.

8. Sit for about 5 minutes the first week or so (try timing yourself with a kitchen timer so that you don't have to keep track of the time). Gradually increase the time you meditate to 15 to 30 minutes a day.

PROGRESSIVE RELAXATION

Progressive relaxation is a technique used to induce nerve-muscle relaxation. It was developed by Edmund Jacobson, M.D., a physician who designed the technique for nervous hospital patients. It involves tensing one muscle group, then relaxing it, slowly moving from one muscle group to another. The purpose of first contracting the muscle is to teach people to recognize more readily what muscle tension feels like—to sense more readily when muscles are tense and then learn to relax them. Progressive relaxation has psychological benefits as well. Studies show that self-esteem is raised, depression lessened, and sleep problems alleviated in people who practice this relaxation method over a period of several weeks.

Usually, a progressive relaxation session begins by tensing then releasing the muscles of the feet and legs, then moves slowly upward, to the hips, abdomen, lower back, upper back, arms, and neck. After you have more experience with progressive relaxation, you should be able to relax individual muscle groups—the muscles of the lower back, for instance, from a standing or seated position. At the start, it may be best to work through your body, from feet to head. The following exercise will help get you started:

Progressive Relaxation Exercise

1. Stretch out on the floor with your knees bent. Make sure that the small of your back is on the floor so that you do not risk straining those muscles. If you like, support your head with a small pillow.

2. Take a deep breath and tighten the muscles of your feet by clenching your toes.
3. As you relax your feet, exhale. Notice the difference in the way your feet feel.
4. Breathe in again, and tighten the muscles of your calves. Hold the exertion for a few seconds.
5. As you exhale and release your calf muscles, say to yourself, "I feel relaxed."
6. Continue the process, with your knees, thighs, stomach, chest, arms, shoulders, lower back, upper back, neck, and face. Each time you tighten and release the muscles, feel yourself sink deeper and deeper into a state of relaxation.
7. When you have finished the process, breathe steadily and deeply for five minutes, enjoying the sense of relaxation.
8. Repeat the exercise daily.

Learning to Relax

As you learn more about your body and the way it reacts to stress, you may be able to attain the relaxed state more quickly and directly. For example, you may be working at your desk and notice that your shoulder muscles are tense. To relax them you can tense them further, and then let them relax. When you focus on the warm, relaxed sensation of your shoulder muscles, you may feel your entire body, and spirit, relax as well.

No matter what method of relaxation you choose, try never to make relaxing seem like a chore, but rather a release and a joy. These simple hints are meant to help you find peace and avoid frustration:

Plan to Relax. When you know a deadline is coming up, or that the week is going to be particularly busy and stressful, try to schedule some time—even just a few minutes—during each day to perform one of the relaxation methods described above or to simply take a walk to relieve the pressure. Chances are, you'll return to the task at hand feeling rejuvenated and better able to focus your attention.

Increase Your Sense of Self-esteem and Control. Learning that you have power and control over your internal environment and realizing that you can make successful, positive changes in your physical and mental health will automatically raise your self-esteem and give you a new sense of self-confidence. With patience and dedication, these habits may well become a favorite part of your daily routine.

Remember to Laugh. Although it may have become a bit of a cliché to say so, laughter truly is one of the best medicines known to man. Humor provides a healthy balance to all the hostility, anxiety, and tension we feel every day. If you can look at the world and yourself with a bit of humor and a touch of whimsy, you'll find that your mind is not as cluttered, your stress is not so great, and your aches and pains less intrusive and debilitating.

The five relaxation methods discussed in this chapter should help you to improve your state of mind and your general health, as well as help to alleviate your back pain. Another often overlooked factor in the development and progression of chronic pain of all kinds is our diet. Indeed, as we'll discuss in Chapter 6, what we eat—or fail to eat—on a daily basis has a direct effect on the state of our physical and emotional health.

"The journey

is the reward."

Tao saying

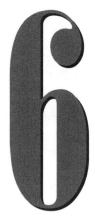

The Diet and Nutrition Factor

$\mathcal{A}$lthough we tend to discuss diet and nutrition in relationship to such diseases as high blood pressure, heart disease, and gastrointestinal disorders, the fact is, what we eat affects every aspect of our physical and emotional selves, including our muscles and bones and our ability to handle stress and tension. If you suffer from back pain, you may well discover that by changing your dietary habits, you'll be helping your body heal itself.

For many Americans, the whole subject of "diet" has become fraught with tedium, frustration, and, more often than not, confusion. One newspaper headline proclaims the virtues of using margarine instead of butter, then—practically the next day—the same newspaper runs a story about the dangers of trans-fatty acids, a common ingredient in margarine. Nevertheless, there are some general prescriptions to follow that will help keep us all on the right path.

In the meantime, it's important to emphasize that the purpose of changing your daily habits is not to add dread or anxiety to your life. As an adult with chronic back pain, you've probably suffered enough of these negative emotions to last a lifetime. Instead, your goal probably should center on adding balance and satisfaction to your daily eating habits, rather than on creating a restrictive or difficult-to-follow diet plan.

One definition of the word balance is "a state of stability, as of the body or the emotions," while another refers to balance as "a state of harmony." By attempting to relieve the symptoms of back pain, you are in essence attempting to reestablish the nutritional, physical, and emotional balance that has been lost in your life.

As you do so, keep in mind that creating a healthy lifestyle should never be a chore to be dreaded or despised. Instead, you should think of it as an opportunity to provide your body and soul with the raw ingredients they need to thrive and flourish. In this chapter, we'll explore four different ways that your diet may be affecting your general health as well as the health of your back:

- Eating to maintain health and strengthen bones and muscles
- Understanding food allergies
- Adding nutritional supplements to your diet
- Learning to enjoy food by establishing relaxing eating patterns

Creating a Balanced Diet

Being overweight is a significant risk factor for the development of back pain. Excess weight can strain back muscles, distort posture, and overly compress the discs in the lower back. Not surprisingly, then, most obese people have chronic back problems. And according to the American Heart Association, more than 170 million Americans are carrying too much weight, which may help to explain why back pain is one of the most common medical complaints in the country today. Why is being overweight so widespread a problem in modern America? Although most of us tend to blame our own lack of willpower and our perceived laziness, we can look to a host of other factors that, over the years, have conspired to turn us into a country of couch potatoes. The preponderance of human energy-saving devices and conveniences, like the automobile, washing machine, and television and VCR, have made it ever so easy to lead a sedentary life.

Think of it this way: At the beginning of this century, more than half of all Americans worked in jobs such as agriculture and construction that met their daily exercise needs. When our great-grandparents and grandparents were growing up, no one joined a health club or took up jogging: They plowed fields, washed clothes by hand, and chopped wood to heat their homes. Even our parents tended to lead more active lives than we do, at least when they were children and adolescents. There were fewer cars, television did not dominate leisure time, and manual labor in the workplace and at home was not so easy to avoid. Today, we have to work at providing our bodies with the cardiovascular and muscular exertion they need to thrive.

At the same time, we grew up at time when the modern supermarket became a warehouse of fat-filled, obesity-inducing substances that we, again over the years, learned to love too much. Vegetables didn't taste good to us unless they were smeared with butter or covered with gravy, fruits were served primarily in sweetened pies, fat-laden meats were favored over fish or vegetable sources of protein, junk food like candy bars and ice cream became staples, and the insistence of convenience over nutrition led to the addition of preservatives, sodium, and other additives to almost every food on grocery store shelves.

Since the 1970s or so, when the so-called health craze hit the United States, we've slowly but surely become more educated about proper nutrition. Unfortunately, because being thin (but not necessarily healthy) in this society has come to represent status and sensuality, the messages about health and fitness have induced anxiety and distress far more often than inspiration and encouragement.

As a result, many of us have developed an unhealthy relationship to food, one that subverts even our best efforts to improve our eating habits. The fact that we've become even more obese in recent years, despite the increased amount of information about nutrition as well as the widespread availability of fat-free foods, is proof of that.

LOSING WEIGHT THROUGH HEALTHY EATING

The attendant anxiety about the state of our bodies creates every bit as much pressure on our backs as any excess poundage we might carry. Therefore, changing our eating habits to reduce the amount of fat and calories (if we need to lose weight) in our diets must be done slowly and with care. Fortunately, the United States Department of Agriculture recently developed an easy-to-understand and healthy eating plan, one that focuses on providing your body with all of the essential nutrients it needs while reducing potentially harmful substances, such as fat and sugar, as much as possible.

The Pyramid Plan, as it is known, is shown on the next page. As you can see, complex carbohydrates (whole-grain bread, pasta, rice, etc.) should make up the bulk of your daily food intake, while fats and sugars should be eaten sparingly. Even without counting calories, it is likely that you'll be able to maintain a healthy weight by following this plan.

On the other hand, if you do need to lose some weight, you'll have to pay even more attention to both what you eat and how much you eat. At the heart of the matter lies this simple fact: To lose weight, you must consume fewer calories than you expend. Since 3,500 calories equal one pound of fat, to lose one pound you must either eat 3,500 fewer calories than your body needs to maintain its weight or burn 3,500 more calories through exercise.

Does losing weight, then, mean eating less and less food? Not necessarily. In fact, studies have shown that active thin people generally take in an average of 600 calories a day *more* than their overweight peers. In this case, the key word is active: These people are working off more calories every day through exercise and the increase in metabolism that regular exercise induces.

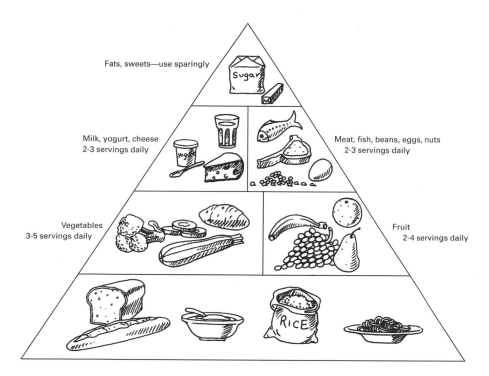

Fats, sweets—use sparingly

Milk, yogurt, cheese
2-3 servings daily

Meat, fish, beans, eggs, nuts
2-3 servings daily

Vegetables
3-5 servings daily

Fruit
2-4 servings daily

Bread, cereal, rice and pasta—6-11 servings daily

The Food Pyramid

*Eating a wholesome diet is an important part of any
prevention and/or treatment plan—mainstream or alternative—for back pain.
Although each individual has his or her own unique dietary needs,
the FDA Food Pyramid, pictured above, offers sound general guidelines
for a healthy, low-fat, high-carbohydrate diet.*

Second, you may be able to eat as much food as you ever have and still lose weight—if you eat the right kind of food. Complex carbohydrates, for instance, are used more efficiently than fat and are therefore less likely to be stored as fat in your body. Also, a gram of fat provides more than twice the calories of a gram of carbohydrates (9 calories compared with 4). That's why one ounce of potato chips—processed in fat and totaling more than 160 calories—is more fattening than one ounce of baked potato, which contains about 30 calories and no fat at all.

In the end, then, you should be able to devise a healthy eating plan that will help you to lose or maintain weight without starving yourself or depriving yourself of satisfying, filling foods. There are many healthy diet plans available, such as those developed by Weight Watchers and the American Heart Association, to guide you through the process if you need additional guidance and support.

FOOD AND ITS IMPACT ON INFLAMMATION

In the meantime, however, there are a few tips we'd like to offer about food and its impact on back pain that go beyond the weight issue. Specifically, certain foods, or substances within food, may either exacerbate or inhibit the inflammatory response—the body's response to injury or infection involving pain, heat, redness, and swelling. (Back injuries that can trigger the inflammatory response include muscle sprains, strains, dislocated discs, among others.)

Later in this chapter, we'll discuss the possibility that a food allergy or sensitivity may be a factor in the development of your particular case of back pain. Even if you do not suffer from a food allergy, you may want to consider reducing certain foods in your diet while increasing the amount you eat of others. In this way, you may be able to relieve some achiness and discomfort, while at the same time strengthening your musculoskeletal system. If you suffer from chronic or acute bouts of back pain, pay attention to the following foods when you consider your diet:

Protein. Protein is found in every body cell, constitutes the second most plentiful substance (after water) in the body of a normal-weight person, and makes up about one fifth of a normal adult's body weight. More important for this discussion, protein is the major component of your muscles and bones. In order for the health of your muscles, tendons, ligaments, and bones to be maintained, you need to consume some protein every day.

Unfortunately, however, Americans tend to eat huge quantities of protein—far more than we need—and most of it comes from high-fat, high-cholesterol sources such as red meat and whole-milk cheese. A diet high in animal protein not only contributes to obesity but may also increase the loss of calcium in the body, which may lead to osteoporosis. In addition, a high-protein diet places enormous strain on the kidneys, which must work to excrete the extra waste products derived from the breakdown of protein.

So although your musculoskeletal health depends on the consumption of sufficient protein, you must guard against eating too much of the wrong kind of this substance. The good news is that protein can be found in a wide variety of foodstuffs, including grains, nuts, beans and lentils, as well as low-fat animal sources such as tuna and other fish, light-meat chicken, and turkey breast.

Your protein prescription: If you eat a normal, balanced diet—one high in complex carbohydrates and low in fat—you can easily provide your body with all the protein it needs. The average man or woman of 150 pounds needs to eat about 55 grams of protein every day. You can obtain that amount by consuming the equivalent of four ounces of white-meat chicken, one cup of pasta, one cup of skim milk, and a half a cup of cooked lima beans.

Fruits and Vegetables. Both fruits and vegetables are, with few exceptions, low in fat and calories, high in fiber, and full of vitamins and minerals. Of most importance in terms of alleviating back pain are the antioxidants found in these foods, specifically beta-carotene (which the body converts to vitamin A), vitamins C and E, and the mineral selenium. Antioxidants appear to reduce the harmful effects of the inflammatory process by protecting muscle, tendon, and ligament cells from being damaged by free radicals—unstable molecules created by various normal chemical processes in the body (like the immune response that causes inflammation) or by environmental influences like radiation and cigarette smoke. The more antioxidants you consume, the less likely there will be damage to your cells.

Your fruit and vegetable prescription: It's fairly safe to say that the more fresh fruit and vegetables you eat, the better. According to the Food Pyramid, you should strive to eat 2 to 4 servings of fresh fruit and 3 to 5 (or more) fresh vegetable servings every day. For more information about how specific vitamins and minerals may affect the inflammatory process, and thus your back pain, see the section "The ABCs of Nutritional Supplements" later in this chapter.

Calcium. Although we tend to think of bones as hard, dead tissue, they are, in fact, very much alive and very active. Bone tissue is constantly taking up and releasing several different minerals to maintain its strength and density. Of primary importance is the mineral calcium, which is the essential factor in building bones and teeth, as well as in helping to produce proper muscle contraction. Without sufficient calcium and other minerals, the process of bone loss known as osteoporosis can take place, especially as we get older. When osteoporosis occurs in the spine and hips, back pain is a frequent side effect.

The body begins to build bone mass in infancy and continues to do so throughout childhood and young adulthood. As you age, however, you need to consume extra calcium because your body no longer absorbs calcium from food as efficiently as it did when you were younger. Furthermore, we tend to eat foods that cause us to excrete too much calcium—substances like sodium, caffeine, and carbonated beverages are especially damaging to the process of calcium absorption.

Although calcium gets the lion's share of attention when it comes to osteoporosis, it is hardly the only mineral necessary to keep your musculoskeletal system healthy. Calcium works best in conjunction with other nutrients, such as vitamin D, magnesium, and boron, among others.

Your calcium prescription: In order to achieve maximum bone density, your body must have a calcium intake high enough to maintain the structural integrity of your bones as well as to compensate for the calcium losses that occur with excretion. Your goal should be to take in about 1,000 milligrams or more of calcium each day—1,500 if you are a pregnant or a woman past the age of menopause. Milk, yogurt, and cheese products have high amounts of easily absorbed calcium, but to avoid consuming too much fat, choose low-fat or skim versions of these foods. In addition, you should try to add nondairy foods rich in calcium, such as sardines and leafy green vegetables (turnip greens, collard greens, and broccoli, for instance) to your diet.

Calcium is not the only nutrient important for the maintenance of healthy bones. You need to consume adequate amounts of vitamin D (found in fish, fortified milk, and also produced in the body in response to sunlight), magnesium (found in whole grains, raw leafy green vegetables, nuts, and bananas), and other nutrients, such as boron and selenium. If you eat a balanced diet, you should be able to attain enough of these vitamins and minerals from the foods you eat. If you have reason to suspect that you aren't getting enough of a certain nutrient, you may want to consider taking a nutritional supplement.

Fats. Although all fat has the potential to make you fat if you eat too much of it, all fat is not alike. While some fats in the diet are crucial to many different body processes, other fats may damage body cells. Generally speaking, animal fat from meat and dairy products will tend to aggravate the inflammatory response—and thus contribute to back pain—while fats derived from cold-water fish such as mackerel, herring, sardines, and salmon will help to reduce inflammation. Fish oils contain a substance called omega-3, which works to stop animal fats from doing damage to cells.

Your fat prescription: According to the American Heart Association and the United States Dietary Association, a healthy diet should derive no more than 30 percent of its calories from fat—any kind of fat. Furthermore, you want to reduce, as much as possible, the amount of saturated fat, such as that found in animal products and hydrogenated vegetable shortenings.

THE SUGAR CONNECTION

Like fat, sugar is a vital substance to the human body. Glucose, the main sugar in the blood and a basic fuel for the body, is essential to the functioning of all cells. But you don't need to consume any sugar at all to supply your body with glucose. Instead, your body breaks down complex carbohydrates (grains, vegetables, and fruits) and sometimes proteins and fats to produce all the glucose it needs.

Whenever you eat food, the hormone insulin is released into the bloodstream. Through a complicated chemical process, insulin helps the cells of the body absorb glucose and use it as energy. Some glucose is stored in the liver and in muscle tissue in the form of glycogen.

When the body needs extra energy during times of physical exertion or emotional stress glycogen is converted into glucose and used as energy.

Some people think that eating sugary foods will boost their energy levels. When we eat simple sugars, such as refined table sugar or the sugar found in cookies and candy, blood glucose levels do rise quickly. But insulin levels rise just as fast and, before you know it, you experience a drop in glucose levels.

Your muscles—including those that support your spine—may become exhausted and thus more likely to become sprained, strained, or otherwise injured.

In addition, a chemical bonding occurs between muscle tissue, joint linings, and the sugar in the fluid that bathes them. This reaction, called glycosylation, goes on continually and irreversibly in direct proportion to the level of sugar in the blood.

Hence, the more bonding that takes place, the more work your body tissues must perform. Therefore, the more sugar you consume, the more quickly your tissues may become damaged through this process.

Finally, excess sugar in your diet and bloodstream may interfere with the proper functioning of your immune system. Should the immune system fail for this reason, infection may occur, further exhausting your body and leaving you open to aches and pain.

Generally speaking, there is no need to deny yourself an occasional sugary indulgence if you have a sweet tooth. However, for many reasons, including those directly related to back pain, you should try to limit the amount of sugar you eat on a daily basis.

Understanding the
Food Allergy Connection

One man's nectar is another's poison—at least when it comes to the food we eat and the way it affects us. Some people are highly sensitive to certain foods, or substances in food, that may worsen their back pain symptoms.

If you have any reason to believe that your case of back pain could be related to osteoarthritis, rheumatoid arthritis, or another inflammatory condition, you may want to ask your doctor about testing for food allergies. There is much evidence to show that the inflammatory response can be triggered in some individuals by an allergic hypersensitivity to certain foods or food-related substances.

An allergy is an immune system reaction to a substance that most people find harmless. Your immune system is designed to defend your body against harmful organisms and substances, such as bacteria, viruses, and other invaders. When the immune system recognizes a substance as being harmful, it mounts a response by producing antibodies and chemicals that attack the offending substance.

If your immune system reacts to generally benign foreign substances, such as pollen, or certain foods, you are allergic to that material. When you come into contact with a food or environmental factor (such as pollen or molds or tobacco smoke) to which you are allergic, your immune system attacks it just as if it were a virus or bacteria. It releases a substance called histamine (a body chemical that can act as an irritating stimulant). When histamine is released in the lungs, it causes secretion of mucus and narrowing and swelling of the lining of the airways. This leads to wheezing and coughing. In some cases, histamine may be released in the joints of the hip and/or spine, which causes an inflammatory response that may result in back pain.

Although you may be allergic to any food, the most common culprits when it comes to back pain, especially back pain related to arthritis, are plants of the nightshade family, including tomatoes, potatoes, eggplant, and peppers. These foods tend to trigger the inflammatory response. Another plant of the nightshade family is tobacco. Not only might tobacco cause an allergic reaction, nicotine has been shown to reduce blood flow to the muscles and spine, further complicating matters for anyone with back pain.

If you are concerned that your symptoms are affected by food or other substances that you consume, talk to your doctor. He or she may suggest that you keep track of your diet and symptoms, writing down the foods you eat, when you eat them, and the symptoms that arise over the course of a day. After a few weeks, a pattern may—or may not—appear. If it appears that your back pain is triggered by a certain food, it would, of course, make sense for you to avoid that food in the future.

In the end, the rule of thumb should be: "If it makes you feel bad, don't eat it!" Instead, eat the foods that contribute to your general health and sense of well-being, and avoid those that appear to intensify your symptoms or otherwise upset your system.

And if you smoke, stop as soon as you can. Talk to your health practitioner about natural herbs, chlorophyll, and the amino acid L-glutamine, which may help you in your effort to beat the habit. Acupuncture, hypnosis, and biofeedback have all been used successfully in stop-smoking programs, but the first step is to sit down and really convince yourself that you want to stop. If you try to quit just because someone tells you its bad for you, you probably won't be successful.

The ABCs of Nutritional Supplements

Although in the best of all possible worlds we would receive all the nutrients we need from the food we eat, many researchers believe that supplementing our diets with certain vitamins and minerals is an important component in any successful treatment of back pain. The following nutrients are those most often mentioned in this connection:

Boron. The trace mineral boron appears to offer several benefits to those who suffer from back pain. It has been shown to have a positive effect on the absorption of calcium into bone, especially in women past the age of menopause. This increased calcium absorption could help to reduce osteoporosis and the back pain it may induce. Some studies show that supplementing your diet every day with about 10 to 20 milligrams (mg) of boron may be beneficial, and is certainly not harmful. In food, boron can be found in high quantities in non-citrus fruits, leafy vegetables, nuts and legumes, wine, and cider.

Vitamin B Complex. All of the B vitamins, including vitamins B_1, B_2, B_3, B_6, B_{12}, and folic acid, are considered important to the healthy development and maintenance of bones and muscle in the body. In addition, vitamins B_1, B_3, and B_6 are particularly helpful in reducing anxiety and thus can help prevent back pain caused by excess stress. Vitamin B_6 has also been shown to help reduce the pain of carpal tunnel syndrome, an impingement of the median nerve of the wrist and strain of the tendons of the hand and shoulder. It is quite possible that vitamin B_6 would also help to alleviate pain caused by similar functional problems in the back.

Foods rich in B vitamins include fish, nuts, grains, eggs, liver, and lean meats. If you and your health practitioner feel you aren't getting enough B vitamins in your diet, you may want to take about 25 to 100 mg of vitamin B complex (available in both a one-dose time-release form or in several smaller doses throughout the day). In addition, if nerve and tendon involvement is suspected, you may want to add a dose of vitamin B_6, up to 10 to 50 mg per day. If you are particularly anxious or under stress, you can add up to 3,000 mg a day of vitamin B_3 (also known as niacin).

Vitamins C, E, and Other Antioxidants. As discussed above, antioxidants help prevent the breakdown of body cells, including that which occurs with exercise. The soreness you may feel after strenuous activity may be due in part to tissue-damaging oxygen molecules generated during exercise. These oxygen molecules attack the fats in muscle cell membranes, weakening the cells and leaving them open to further injury.

In addition, prolonged or muscle-damaging exercise triggers the immune system to respond in much the same way as it does to infection, in essence launching an attack to break down the damaged muscle tissue so that new tissue can replace the old. The attack may get out of control and thus damage healthy muscle tissue as well. Antioxidants, especially vitamin E, have been found to effectively slow down this process.

By increasing the amount of antioxidants you eat in fresh fruit and vegetables, as well as by taking vitamin supplements, you can thus help prevent your back muscle cells from becoming damaged, inflamed, and sore. Recommended dosages of vitamin C supplements range from 250 to 3,000 mg per day. Please note, however, vitamin C can be quite acidic—the more you take, the more risk you have for developing stomach irritation. Recommended dosages of vitamin E supplements range from 200 to 800 international units (IU) per day.

Omega-3 Fatty Acids. These fatty acids, derived mainly from cold-water fish such as mackerel and salmon, inhibit the inflammatory response. (In addition, omega-3 also helps to reduce cholesterol levels in the body.) If you wish to supplement your diet, you can take up to 1,000 to 10,000 mg per day. Make sure you purchase supplements that contain 150 to 1,000 mg of EPA, the active fatty acid in this substance.

Magnesium. As well as working with calcium to help form strong and healthy bones, magnesium plays an important role in muscle contraction and relaxation. Magnesium also is required for the production of a body chemical called adenosine triphosphate (ATP), the molecular "power cell" on which the body depends to perform nearly all of its physical, mental, and biochemical work.

Magnesium is found in high quantities in green leafy vegetables, nuts, and legumes. However, many of us may not get enough magnesium, particularly women who take birth control pills, heavy drinkers, and people whose diets consist primarily of refined foods. You can take magnesium supplements of up to 600 to 800 mg a day to compensate for this deficiency or to bolster the supply you receive from fresh foods.

DL-Phenylalanine. Also known as DLPA, this man-made amino acid supplement has been shown to be an effective pain reliever because it appears to inhibit the breakdown of endorphins, thereby increasing the effect of these components of the body's own pain-relieving system.

THE DIET AND NUTRITION FACTOR

Selenium. This trace mineral is a component of an enzyme that is responsible for preventing the buildup of free radicals. By taking just 200 micrograms of this nutrient every day, you can help protect your muscles and bones from becoming damaged. Please note that selenium does not work alone: It requires sufficient amounts of vitamin E to function efficiently as an antioxidant.

Now that you've read about how to improve your diet by avoiding foods that may be harmful to your health while bolstering your own internal health-promoting faculties, it's time to address another important issue: The way you think about eating may be affecting your levels of stress and thus your state of tension and anxiety on a daily basis.

Establish a Healthy Approach to Eating

Food is nourishment. The nutrients in the food you eat every day are the catalysts for millions of major and minor miracles—the beating of your heart, the birth of an idea, the appreciation of taste and smell—that take place within the chemistry lab that is your body.

Food is also a source of pleasure. We do not eat merely to ingest the various vitamins, minerals, and other substances we need to survive. Instead, eating is a supremely sensual activity: We smell food's aromas, taste its flavors, admire its colors and textures, and feel its consistency inside our mouths. Depending on the circumstances, our sense of hearing may be equally stimulated by the conversation of our tablemates or the sounds of soothing dinner music.

As you consider your dietary habits, ask yourself these questions: Do you take the time to enjoy the sensual aspects of eating, or do you simply think of food as fuel for the body? Or conversely, do you eat only those things that taste good without considering their nutritional value? Are there foods that you enjoy eating but which seem to exacerbate your back pain or otherwise upset your system? Depending on how you answer these questions, you may discover that your approach to eating could use a little readjustment.

RULES TO EAT BY

As you structure an eating plan that's right for you, keep in mind these general goals:

All good things in moderation. Unless you have a specific allergy or sensitivity, it appears that no food is off-limits for you in terms of coping with back pain. However, in order to maintain a healthy and fit body and mind, limit the amount of fat, sugar, caffeine, and alcohol you consume on a regular basis.

Add variety to your diet. By eating lots of different kinds of food during the day, not only will you improve your chances of getting all the nutrients you need, you'll also probably find yourself enjoying your diet more than ever before. At least once a week, make it a point to try a new food—an exotic fruit or vegetable, for instance—or cook a different dish.

Take time to enjoy the sensual aspects of eating. Too often we find ourselves gulping down food without really tasting its flavors or enjoying its textures and aromas. Eating food on the run also means denying ourselves the pleasure of setting an elegant table and lingering over a fine meal in the company of family and friends. Try to take the time to make eating an experience to be savored rather than an automatic activity.

Plan special meals and treats. Although we should all aim to eat healthy, wholesome foods as often as possible, many of us have cravings for foods that are less than ideal—and we should never try to permanently deprive ourselves of these foods. By building some occasional indulgences into our diets, we can satisfy those cravings without undermining our otherwise healthy eating plans. Depending on your weight, health, and personal tastes, you might want to plan to eat a special dessert once a week or a cheeseburger lunch with all the trimmings once a month.

Eat foods that leave you feeling healthy and well. Pay attention to how you feel after you eat your meals. If you're often groggy and uncomfortable, you may be eating too much, failing to eat a balanced diet, or consuming food that doesn't agree with your particularly body makeup. Nutritious food, prepared well, and eaten in a relaxed atmosphere should nourish your body and your soul. If you need further information, talk to your doctor or a nutritionist.

You've now had a chance to see how what you eat may affect your muscles, bones, and emotional life. In the next chapter, we take a look at another approach to alleviating back pain, one that focuses on the healing powers of the human hands on injured, painful muscles and joints.

"Nature
heals, the doctor
nurses."

Anonymous

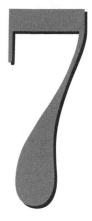

Hands-on Help:
Bodywork
and Massage

....

*T*he human touch is perhaps the most underrated therapy for the relief of back pain, headaches, and a host of other stress-related and musculoskeletal problems in this country. Our modern medical doctors tend to favor high-tech diagnostic and therapeutic techniques over the more subtle and intuitive methods of touch and one-to-one communication.

Even in our personal lives, we Americans are inclined to keep our hands to ourselves. A study conducted in the 1960s compared the touching behaviors of pairs of people sitting in coffee shops around the world. In San Juan, Puerto Rico, people touched 180 times an hour; in Paris, France, they touched an average of 110 times an hour, while in Gainesville, Florida, people touched each other just twice every hour.

By avoiding touching one another, we are missing out on one of the most meaningful forms of human communication and one of the most effective therapeutic methods known to man. How can touch do so much? Consider this: Your skin is one of your largest and most important organs, covering about 12 to 19 square feet and weighing between 5 and 8 pounds, depending upon your height and weight. In addition to forming a protective sheath around your muscles, blood vessels, and internal organs, your skin is an extremely sensitive and animate structure. A piece of skin about an inch in size contains more than 3 million cells, 100 to 300 sweat glands, 3 feet of blood vessels, and more than 50 nerve endings.

It should come as no surprise, then, that when your skin is touched, the feelings generated reach far below the surface into the very depths of your emotional self. And when stronger pressure is applied, your muscles, tissues, and organs benefit.

For centuries, healers from virtually every culture around the world have used the power of touch as a method of curing illness and relieving pain. In recent decades, massage and other methods of bodywork using the human hands as instruments of health and healing have finally been gaining in popularity and acceptance across the United States as well.

In this chapter, we discuss some of the ways that bodywork techniques can help to heal the body and bring it closer to the ideal state of balance and integrity we know as health. Performed by expert hands, massage is able to

- Help relax the body by calming the nervous system
- Soothe tense and cramped muscles
- Break up scar tissue and loosen adhesions that may form after injury to muscles or long periods of inactivity
- Foster healing by stimulating circulation of immune system cells
- Trigger the release of endorphins, the body's natural painkillers
- Increase blood flow, helping to remove harmful chemical waste products from muscle and nerve tissue
- Help reduce swelling and other symptoms of inflammation

- Release pent-up, potentially toxic emotions through deep breathing and verbal expression during massage
- Bring the muscles, bones, connective tissue, and organs back into proper alignment

There are virtually dozens of different bodywork and massage techniques from which to choose. Although the goal of all forms of massage and bodywork is to return the body to a balanced, healthy state, each technique is slightly different. Below is a brief overview of several different methods available in the United States today. You can find out even more about them by calling or writing the organizations and agencies listed under "Bodywork and Massage" in *Natural Resources*, page 188.

Therapeutic Massage

The word *massage* is derived from the Arabic *massa*, which means to stroke. Therapeutic massage and its offshoot Swedish massage involve kneading and stroking the skin and applying pressure on tense muscles. Tapping, clapping, or similar percussive hand movements along the spine and muscles may also be employed.

Developed in Sweden about 150 years ago, Swedish massage is the most popular form in the United States. The technique involves five basic strokes:

- *Effleurage* consists of long, gliding strokes from the neck down to the base of the spine or from the shoulder down to the fingertips. Effleurage is designed to acquaint the therapist with his or her subject's body and vice versa.
- *Petrissage* involves gently lifting muscles up and away from the bones, then rolling and squeezing them, again with a gentle pressure. Petrissage attempts to increase circulation with clearing out toxins from muscle and nerve tissue.

- *Friction* strokes consist of applying deep, circular movement near joints and other bony areas (such as the sides of the spine) with thumbs and fingertips. Friction breaks down adhesions, which are knots that result when muscle fibers bind together during the healing process, thus contributing to more flexible muscles and joints.
- *Tapotement* is a short chopping stroke applied in several different ways: with the edge of the hand, with the tips of the fingers, or with a closed fist. Tapotement attempts to release tension and cramping from muscles in spasm.
- *Vibration*, or shaking, involves the therapist pressing his or her hands on your back or limbs, and rapidly shaking for a few seconds. Meant to boost circulation and increase the power of the muscles to contact, vibration is particularly helpful to people suffering from low-back pain.

Many health professionals now practice massage, including physical therapists, athletic trainers, nurses, as well as licensed or certified massage therapists. A visit to a massage therapist typically lasts from 30 to 60 minutes. In most cases, you will be asked to remove your clothing, lie down on a massage table, and drape a sheet or towel over your body. Before he or she begins the session, the therapist may ask about your medical history and current emotional and physical state. Your privacy and modesty should be respected at all times by the therapist. Pleasantly scented oils may be used during the massage.

In addition to Western forms of therapeutic massage, of which there are any number of variations, there exist Eastern massage techniques, primarily *shiatsu* and *acupressure,* both of which developed out of Chinese medical theory. According to Chinese medicine, we have energy channels, called meridians, which run through the body and through which energy flows. When energy becomes blocked, pain and disease may occur. In Chapter 9, Chinese Medicine and Back Pain, the philosophy and techniques of shiatsu and acupressure will be discussed in some detail. For now, it is enough to say that these widely used methods of massage focus on releasing energy that has become blocked within the body while at the same time applying healing, soothing massage.

The Alexander Technique

Posture—the way we hold our body as we stand, sit, and move—has a direct effect on the state of our physical and mental health, or so claimed Frederick Matthias Alexander, a turn-of-the-century Australian Shakespearean actor. Plagued by chronic voice loss, Alexander studied the way he spoke by reciting his lines in front of a mirror. What he noticed surprised him: Whenever he began to speak, or even thought of speaking, he tended to tense his neck, move his head back and forth, and slightly hunch his back. When he altered these habitual muscular movements, however, he found that his voice returned in full strength.

Based on his own experience, Alexander put forward the theory that the root cause of many disorders—especially those directly connected to the musculoskeletal system such as back pain—is the muscular tension that results from holding our bodies in the wrong position over many years. He developed a technique by which practitioners could help subjects "unlearn" faulty movements or postures.

The heart of the Alexander Technique consists of allowing your spine to slowly stretch upward to its optimal length by releasing the tension in your neck and lifting your head up so it sits just above the spine. Whenever you move, you should lead with your head, follow with the spine, and let your body lengthen to its full, balanced extent.

During a typical Alexander Technique session, which can last up to an hour and a half, you might be asked to sit, stand, or lie on a table (fully clothed). The practitioner will then touch your head, neck, and spine, feeling for any tension or muscular compression. Gently, the practitioner will move your body into alignment, helping you with words and motion to find your correct posture and release your back and neck muscles. Eventually, over time, you will have learned to hold and move your body in a whole new and, hopefully, pain-free way.

Today, there are about 500 teachers of the Alexander Technique nationwide. To be affiliated with the national professional society—the North American Society of Teachers of the Alexander Technique—a practitioner must have completed at least 1,600 hours of training.

The Feldenkrais Method

According to Moshe Feldenkrais, your case of back pain may well be caused by negative patterns of movement resulting from your own self-image, a self-image that induces you to hold your body in a certain way as you go through your day. If you want to change the way your back feels, Feldenkrais theory postulates, you have to change the way you think about yourself and about the way you move.

Like the Alexander technique, the Feldenkrais Method attempts to break old habits and replace them with new ones. If you visit a Feldenkrais practitioner, referred to as a "teacher," you will be asked to lie down on a table (fully clothed) or sit upright in a chair. The teacher very gently moves different parts of your body, showing you and telling you how your body is meant to move, freely and in balance. Instead of forcing a particular posture upon your body, the Feldenkrais Method helps you explore and experiment until you find the style of movement that makes you feel strong and centered, and free from pain.

About 300 practitioners are certified in the Feldenkrais Method in the United States today. In about three years of part-time study, they learn how to recognize misalignments and imbalances, and work with individuals to reverse them.

Myotherapy

A technique developed by Bonnie Prudden, myotherapy is based on the idea that past injuries can result in hidden pockets of pain called "trigger points." Trigger points can be caused by any trauma—emotional or physical—at any age and in any part of the body. Trigger points related to back pain may involve old strains or sprains caused by an accident, by years of poor posture, or by any of a number of emotional wounds and scars. Once activated, trigger points force the affected muscle to shorten and remain that way, restricting its range of motion.

When you visit a myotherapist, he or she will first take a medical history and ask you about your symptoms. You will then be asked to remove your clothes and put on a gown. Carefully, and using a combination of intuition and training, the therapist will locate your trigger points by gently pressing down upon your back or other body part. Because trigger points can "refer" pain to a distant site in the body along predictable patterns, you shouldn't be surprised if your therapist begins to work on your foot or hand first.

Once a trigger point is found, the therapist will apply pressure to the area directly above a trigger point using his or her elbow, knuckles, or fingers. Although the subject often feels pain with the pressure, once the pressure is released, the pain disappears. Because a slight soreness may remain for a day or two as the muscles released try to rewind themselves into their old, tensed positions, the therapist may suggest various stretching exercises and massage techniques you can perform yourself.

In order to receive treatment from a myotherapist, you must be referred by a physician. There are about 200 certified myotherapists practicing in the country today.

Rolfing

This technique, also called *structural integration,* was developed in the 1970s by Ida Rolf, a biochemist. According to Dr. Rolf, pain and disease occur when the body comes out of proper alignment through habitual poor posture and movement. Over time, the fascia (the connective tissue covering muscles and organs) has to compensate and stretch to hold everything in this incorrect and eventually painful position. As this occurs, the fascia becomes more rigid and solid as adhesions, or scarring, occurs.

In order to return the body to health and balance, Dr. Rolf suggested that the deep connective tissue be manipulated and stretched back into place. As the fascia returned to its natural position, the muscles, blood vessels, and nerves that had been out of alignment would slowly work themselves back into place. Finally, the body would be remade to conform to its original design, forming one single vertical line extending from the head and shoulders through the thorax and down into the legs. When this occurs, posture improves, muscles work more easily and with more strength, and self-esteem is elevated.

Rolfing, as this technique is called, is not painless. In order to stimulate and realign deep connective tissue, the Rolfer (the therapist) must apply some force as he or she massages tissues. It is likely that at your first visit to a Rolfer, your photograph will be taken so that you can see the way you hold your body as you stand and sit. You'll be asked about your medical history, your emotional state, and your back pain and other current symptoms. You will then lie down on a table or the floor (fully clothed or in your underwear) while the Rolfer works through your body, kneading your joints and muscles with his or her fingers, knuckles, or elbows. In this way, the Rolfer intends to reorganize the fascial tissue back into its proper alignment and lifting, lengthening, and balancing the body.

Rolfers receive training at the Rolf Institute in Boulder, Colorado. The course involves two nine-week training sessions, followed by a series of continuing education classes after certification.

The Trager Approach and Zero-Balancing

Milton Trager, M.D., devised this unique form of bodywork more than 50 years ago. By rocking, shaking, and stretching your body—ever so gently—a Trager practitioner attempts to bring an individual's body into a more natural and relaxed state. Practitioners do so not only by massaging the body but by attempting to release negative patterns that subjects hold within their mind. Such a process is extraordinarily personal and intuitive on the part of both the practitioner and the person receiving treatment.

In addition to hands-on bodywork, the Trager approach also teaches Mentastics, simple, free-flowing movements designed to increase your awareness of how your body moves now and, most important, how you can allow it to move more effortlessly. For someone with lower-back pain, the "slow pendulum movement" Mentastic exercise is often recommended. In this exercise, you stand up and slowly shift your weight to the right foot, then back over to the left foot. Subtle and simple, this movement helps to heighten awareness of your body's innate symmetry and alignment and thus bring it back into balance.

A Trager session lasts about an hour and a half. Most people visit a Trager practitioner once a week, perhaps more when acute back pain is involved. Trager therapists undergo six months to one year of specialized training in the Trager approach. Because of the intimate, intuitive nature involved in the Trager approach, a good and trusting relationship between you and the practitioner is essential.

A related discipline, called Zero-balancing and created by California osteopath Fritz Smith, is a simple technique involving gentle realignment of the spine.

Some General Precautions

Although these methods of bodywork and massage are safe for most people, it is important that you follow a few general suggestions before you visit a massage therapist of any kind:

Get a thorough medical evaluation of your back pain problem. The cause of most cases of back pain cannot be identified, and for the majority of these individuals, bodywork may help to alleviate the condition. However, there are some cases in which massage or bodywork can do more harm than good, especially if deep massage is performed. Certain types of disc fractures or herniations, for instance, may worsen with massage. Talk to your doctor or practitioner about your particular problem before making a massage appointment.

Do not receive a massage when you are suffering from a high fever or another infectious or malignant condition. Because massage stimulates blood flow, bacteria, viruses, and even cancer cells may—

in certain cases—spread more quickly throughout the body if you undergo massage therapy. Again, talk to your doctor or practitioner if you have any questions.

Massage may not be for you if you suffer from varicose veins, phlebitis, or other blood vessel problems. Vigorous massage could further stress vessels or even dislodge a blood clot.

Make sure the massage or bodywork therapist you choose is qualified. In *Natural Resources*, page 188, we provide a list of agencies and public service centers that will be happy to refer you to trained and certified professionals. If you have any question about your therapist's qualifications, check with one of these associations.

"The great art

of life

is sensation,

to feel

that we exist,

even in pain."

Lord Byron

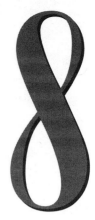

Spinal Manipulation: Chiropractic and Osteopathy

*J*n 1992, a Rand Corporation study revealed that spinal manipulation—the chief tool of two forms of alternative medicine known as chiropractic and osteopathy—surpassed surgery and drugs for the relief of back pain in most people. The Rand study confirmed a great deal of other previous research, including a 1990 report in the *British Journal of Medicine,* showing that spinal manipulation therapy was far more successful than conventional medicine in treating back pain.

In essence, spinal manipulation therapy is just what it sounds like: treatment of back pain and other disorders involving readjusting the vertebrae. As discussed in Chapter 3, the spinal column is made up of 24 bones called vertebrae that surround the spinal cord, which is a sheaf of nerve tissue reaching from the base of the skull to the upper part of the lower back. Between adjoining vertebrae are pairs of spinal nerves that extend to every part of the body. Should the vertebrae become misaligned—through trauma, stress, or a chemical imbalance—pressure is placed on the nerves in the affected area. Chronic back pain, as well as a host of other conditions, may be the result.

Two alternative schools of medicine, chiropractic and osteopathy, consider the spine and the nervous system that springs from it to be the center of all health in the body.

Today, more than 94 percent of all manipulative care is delivered by chiropractors, 4 percent by osteopaths, and the remaining 2 percent by general practitioners and orthopedic surgeons. In this chapter, we'll discuss the benefits of chiropractic and osteopathic techniques on lower-back problems.

Chiropractic Technique

Chiropractic is a word derived from the Greek *cheir,* meaning "hand," and *praktikis,* meaning "practical." Although spinal adjustment has been practiced by every culture in recorded history, the modern school of chiropractic was first developed in 1895 by Daniel David Palmer, a self-educated healer. Palmer's first patient was a janitor who had been deaf for almost twenty years. By bringing the man's spine back into alignment through massage and pressure, Palmer restored his hearing. Palmer believed that the janitor had lost his hearing because an injury had damaged his spine, preventing the central nervous system from delivering messages to and from the brain and ear. Palmer also believed that the body had an innate ability to heal itself, an ability controlled by the central nervous system. If the spine became misaligned, then the body could no longer restore balance on its own to any part of the body.

Chiropractic therapy centers on restoring proper balance and structure to the spinal column and joints and, by doing so, restoring proper working order to the nervous system that radiates from the spinal cord to the organs and tissues of the body. When the vertebrae are properly aligned and the spine remains flexible, nerve impulses from the brain can travel freely along the spinal cord and to the all the organs and tissues of the body.

By keeping the spine in alignment through regular visits to the chiropractor, so the theory holds, you will not only help to soothe your current back pain, but also protect your back from further injury. Furthermore, by keeping the nervous system in good working order, you'll be allowing your body to function well as a whole, and thus be able to heal itself of most ailments. According to theory, then, chiropractic can be seen as treatment for injury and pain as well as a method of preventing disease.

BACK TIP

Housecleaning without Pain

- Purchase a duster with an extra-long pole or make one yourself by wrapping a towel around the head of a long-handled broom. That way, you can avoid bending down to sweep dust from beneath radiators or in hard-to-reach corners.

- Never vacuum when you're in pain, and never for more than 15 minutes at a stretch if you suffer from chronic back pain.

- Organize your kitchen so that heavy pots and pans and other commonly used items are kept in cabinets or on counters that are about waist-high.

- Never bend over to clean a toilet or bathtub. Kneel instead.

- If all else fails, hire a maid to come in to clean once or twice a week; a maid is far less expensive in the long run than weeks of bed rest or the cost of physical rehabilitation.

CHIROPRACTIC DIAGNOSIS AND TREATMENT

Your evaluation with a chiropractor begins the minute you walk through the office door. The chiropractor will pay just as much careful attention to the way you walk, stand, and sit as he or she will to any x-ray or other diagnostic test. After watching the way you move, the chiropractor will ask you questions about your symptoms and past medical history. (In fact, because a chiropractor is not a medical doctor, it is extremely important that you rule out any medical problems that could be causing your back pain—such as gastrointestinal disorders, cancer, or other serious conditions—before you visit a chiropractor.) He or she will ask about any recent injuries that may have caused or exacerbated your back pain. Some time will be spent assessing your work, exercise, and nutritional habits to see how they might be contributing to your problem.

Following this discussion, the chiropractor will administer an orthopedic exam, during which special attention is paid to the range of movement of your spine and limbs. You'll probably be asked to bend forward, backward, and sideways, and to rotate your spine. A neurological examination, including reflex testing, is done to assess nerve function. Then the chiropractor may feel the spine and various other joints with his or her hands to further assess mobility and alignment. Under certain circumstances, x-rays may be required to derive more information or to confirm a diagnosis.

Once your chiropractor decides where your particular misalignment—or *subluxation,* as chiropractors term a disturbance in the spine—is, the chiropractic *adjustment* begins. Depending on the kind of subluxation found in your spine, the chiropractor may choose to perform an *active* manipulation, in which you'll be asked to stretch your body in a certain way yourself, or a *passive* manipulation, in which the chiropractor assists your movement, helping to stretch the spine past its range of passive movement using his or her hands. Another process, known as the *high-velocity thrust,* involves the chiropractor placing his or her hands on a particular vertebral area and then thrusting forward with a certain amount of force and speed.

One of the most common chiropractic manipulations used to alleviate low-back pain is called the *side posture adjustment*. If your chiropractor decides this adjustment might help you, you will be asked to lie face down on a padded table, then move slowly onto your left side. Taking your right leg in one hand, the chiropractor will bring it up and over to the left so that it lies near your chest. With his or her other hand, the chiropractor will gently push down on your right shoulder, bringing it as close to the right side of the table as possible. Twisting your waist and lower back in this way allows muscle tension to be released and vertebrae to gently move back into proper position. After holding you in this position for a few minutes, the chiropractor will remove his or her hands and allow your body to return to its side position. You'll then slowly turn onto your right side and repeat the adjustment from this position.

The adjustment chosen and technique used are determined by the chiropractor based on your particular needs and physical constitution. Do not be alarmed if your body makes some cracking or hissing noises: these are signs that the bones are moving and gases within the joints are being released. Although chiropractic should never be painful, you may feel a certain pressure and achiness during and for a few days following your first few treatments.

Appointments usually last from 30 to 60 minutes. Most chiropractors will suggest one or two visits a week for a couple of weeks, then one every three weeks for maintenance. Generally speaking, the more entrenched and long-standing your back problem is, the longer it will take to resolve. On the other hand, if chiropractic is going to work for you, you should see a substantial improvement in symptoms in about a month to six weeks.

FINDING A QUALIFIED CHIROPRACTOR

Chiropractic now ranks as the second-largest primary health care field in the world, with more than 18 million Americans visiting a chiropractor every year, a great majority of them seeking relief from stubborn, chronic back pain. Today, there are more than 50,000 chiropractors practicing in the United States.

Although not medical doctors, chiropractors are among the more highly trained alternative caregivers, requiring at least six years of undergraduate and postgraduate training at colleges accredited by an agency officially recognized by the United States Department of Education. Chiropractors become licensed in all 50 states after passing rigorous state-controlled examinations.

To find a qualified chiropractor, your first step might be to ask your own family doctor. In recent years, chiropractors have been able to form cordial working relationships with much of the mainstream medical community. Also, feel free to ask your friends and acquaintances for referrals—word of mouth is one of the best ways to find a qualified and caring health professional—or check with the American Chiropractic Association or the International Chiropractors Association (see *Natural Resources*, page 188, for more information).

Osteopathy

Although this branch of Western medicine remains new to many Americans, it was founded by a traditional American physician, Andrew Taylor Still, more than 120 years ago. Andrew Still modeled his philosophy of medicine on the theories postulated by the Greek father of medicine, Hippocrates. Hippocrates believed that the body could cure itself and that a doctor should be trained to study aspects of health rather than symptoms of illness in order to understand and treat disease.

In addition, Dr. Still postulated that the body can function properly only if blood and nerve impulses are allowed to flow throughout the body unimpeded. If your spine or another joint comes out of alignment and blocks blood and nerve flow, disease and pain may result. Furthermore, because the musculoskeletal system is the body's largest energy user, tension or restriction in this system can deplete the rest of the body of its energy and thus result in illness.

Of all the medical specialties, osteopathy is considered the most holistic, tending as it does to treat the whole person rather than one set of symptoms or health concerns. Osteopathic treatment centers on restoring balance and order to the musculoskeletal system—and thus to your whole body—through spinal manipulation. Attention is also paid to diet, exercise, and other habits that may be affecting your health.

YOUR OSTEOPATHIC EXAM AND TREATMENT

Unlike chiropractors, osteopaths are licensed medical doctors who receive extra training in spinal manipulation and the musculoskeletal system. Osteopaths are able to perform extensive diagnostic tests, prescribe drugs, and perform surgery. Although most osteopaths are general practitioners, some may have chosen training in a mainstream specialty, such as gynecology, pediatrics, or surgery. In fact, not all osteopaths practice manipulation today, but rather rely completely on mainstream techniques.

Your first appointment with an osteopath should be similar to one with a mainstream physician, with a few notable exceptions. First, an osteopath will most likely spend a great deal of time discussing your general health, your medical history, your symptoms, and your personal habits. Second, he or she will pay special attention to the way you sit, stand, and walk, and may ask you to perform special exercises to see how your body moves. Asymmetry, a condition in which one side of your body is being held off-center, thus placing stress on that part of the body, is one thing osteopaths attempt to identify. Osteopaths also look for any abnormal increase or decrease in the normal curve of the spine.

Third, the osteopath will probably spend far more time touching your body, particularly your spine and lower back, than a mainstream physician might. He or she will feel for temperature and texture changes of the skin, areas of muscular tension, tenderness, or swelling, and nerve reflexes. In some cases, x-rays or MRI studies may be suggested, depending on what the osteopath finds during the initial examination.

Once the source of your problem is located, the osteopath will help you work out a treatment plan. In most cases of back pain, this will involve the following:

- *Medication or surgery:* Because osteopathy blends conventional with alternative approaches, most osteopaths may be more likely than other holistic practitioners to recommend mainstream medical solutions. At the same time, they are more willing to explore other approaches before suggesting surgery.
- *Manipulation:* Like chiropractors, osteopaths use their hands— and sometimes gentle currents of electricity or ultrasound technology—to release tension from muscles and restore proper alignment of the spine and other joints.
- *Relaxation techniques:* By prescribing specially designed exercises and visualization techniques (such as those described in Chapter 5), osteopaths help you to maintain your body's structural integrity by preventing stress and tension from disrupting your musculoskeletal system.
- *Breathing exercises:* Deep breathing exercises are meant to help bring life-enhancing oxygen and other nutrients to all the tissues of the body, as well as to stretch the muscles of the chest and upper and lower back to their full range.
- *Posture correction:* Borrowing from a variety of bodywork techniques, including some of those described in Chapter 7, osteopaths attempt to correct postural imbalances that may be contributing to your case of back pain. By teaching you how to use your body in a more efficient and less stressful way, osteopaths hope to help you reduce the stress and tension that may damage the joints and soft tissue of your back.
- *Nutritional guidance:* Because osteopathy is essentially a holistic approach to health and healing, your osteopath will assess the state of your diet and help you to develop an eating and nutritional plan that will keep you healthy and your back strong.

FINDING A QUALIFIED OSTEOPATH

Today, more than 35,000 osteopaths practice in the United States. The training they receive in the fifteen osteopathic medical colleges blends conventional medical and surgical techniques with osteopathic manipulative techniques. Medical doctors (M.D.s) who are also osteopaths carry the title Doctor of Osteopathy, or D.O., and are listed in the telephone book under "Physicians and Surgeons." See *Natural Resources*, page 188, for more information.

Both chiropractic and osteopathy are largely based on Western medical traditions. In the next chapter, we explore an approach to health and healing that arises from the East, one that embraces some concepts and techniques that may be unfamiliar to you.

"Use the
light that is
within you
to regain your
natural clearness
of sight."

Lao-Tzu

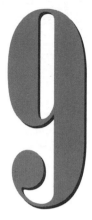

Chinese Medicine and Back Pain

....

*D*iana Westenberg had suffered from chronic low-back pain *for months. The pain tended to get worse whenever the weather was damp, when she was tired, when she ate too much sugar, and sometimes for no apparent reason at all. For many months, she had been taking antiinflammatory drugs on a regular basis, especially around her period. Although they took the edge off the pain, they made her stomach feel queasy. Diana also had regular massages, which also helped make her back feel better, but only for a few hours.*

Desperate for a more lasting solution, Diana decided to try acupuncture, a healing therapy of Chinese medicine. The acupuncturist was someone Diana knew socially, and she was surprised to feel like she was in an exotic environment when she entered the practitioner's office. There were Oriental charts of acupuncture pathways, called meridians, on the walls, and the air smelled vaguely of incense, a smell the acupuncturist told her was moxa, an herb burned as part of some acupuncture treatments.

The acupuncturist took a complete history of Diana's medical condition, her current symptoms (not limited to her back problem), and back pain treatments she had tried in the past. She also asked Diana what seemed like strange questions, including what she considered her favorite foods and her favorite season of the year, whether she liked to be touched on the back, whether warmth or cold made her feel better, and what things made her angry or fearful.

The acupuncturist's examination also included looking at and carefully poking her back in order to find any tender spots. She also examined the belly, again looking for tender spots as well as temperature differences, and inspected the tongue. Finally, the acupuncturist spent a long time taking Diana's pulse, using several fingers to feel the pulse on both wrists.

Diana was then shown a chart on the wall. The acupuncturist explained to her that the examination revealed an energy channel in her body called the "bladder channel" was not functioning properly and was responsible for her back pain. In Chinese medicine, the practitioner explained, the bladder is responsible for holding reserves, not only of urine but of energy, strength, and courage as well. Diana was using up her reserves too quickly, affecting the bladder channel and leading to back pain. A problem like this in the bladder channel could also lead to the need to frequently urinate and a crash of energy in the afternoon. Upon reflection, Diana realized she often experienced both of these symptoms.

The acupuncturist suggested treatment consisting of using small needles placed in tender points along the back. First, she used moxas to warm up these points, then carefully inserted the needles. Other acupuncture points were found in Diana's hands and feet. The procedure wasn't at all painful, although Diana felt a distinct electrical sensation when the needles hit the points.

Slowly but surely, over the course of a few weeks, Diana felt her back pain disappear. She still noticed that using up her energy by staying out late or enduring periods of stress tended to bring on her backaches. She was pleased to see that her energy was not crashing in the afternoon as readily as it had in the past. Regular acupuncture treatments became an important part of her strategy to deal with her backaches, as well as other aspects of her health.

BACK TIP

Make Love, Not Strain

Believe it or not, making love is a great form of exercise; it can help tone the back muscles and release general tension from the body.

However, if you suffer from chronic back pain, certain sexual positions may be more difficult to perform than others. The traditional "missionary position," for instance, puts terrific pressure on a woman's spine and pelvis and on a man's lower back. Instead, experiment with other less stressful positions, such as "two spoons," in which you and your partner lie on your sides with knees drawn up toward the stomach, just like two spoons would fit one inside the other. Backs are supported and movement is not as vigorous or forceful. No matter what position you choose, try to make this time with your partner as comfortable, loving, and stress-free as possible; if you need more advice, talk to your physician or practitioner.

Chinese Medicine:
An Age-Old Philosophy of Health

The acupuncture treatments Diana Westenberg received for her back pain are just one aspect of an ancient medical system developed in China at least 3,000 years ago. Its tenets were recorded in a text called *The Yellow Emperor's Classic of Internal Medicine* more than 2,500 years ago. Millions of people all over the world rely on these principles to keep them healthy and vital today.

Like Diana, you may be most familiar Chinese medicine because of its relationship to acupuncture, which has been widely practiced as a method of pain relief in the United States since the early 1970s. But Chinese medicine involves far more than acupuncture. To truly treat the whole body and bring it back into the state of balance we know of as health, Chinese medicine also relies on herbal medicine and an exercise system known as qi-gong, which will be described later in the chapter.

In the meantime, we'll provide you with a bit of background on the philosophy of Chinese medicine and health. Although it is not essential for you to completely understand or believe in its principles, it may be helpful for you to have an overview of the theories behind the treatment an acupuncturist or Chinese herbalist might use to help alleviate your back pain.

YIN-YANG: THE BALANCE OF LIFE'S ENERGY

At its heart, the Chinese philosophy of health is based on the view that humanity, and each individual human, is part of a larger creation—the universe itself. Each of us is subject to the same laws that govern all of nature. In fact, Chinese medicine refers to the flow of bodily fluid and energy as channels and rivers, and the state of the body as a whole in terms of the natural elements. Don't be surprised if your condition is referred to as "damp" or "dry" or connected to the "water" or "wood" element.

In Chinese medicine, your health is determined by your ability to maintain a balanced and harmonious internal environment. Internal harmony is expressed through the principle of *yin-yang*, in which two opposing forces have united to create everything in the universe. Yin has connotations of cold, dark, and wet, while yang is warm, bright, and dry. Yin is quiet, static, and inactive, while yang is dynamic, active, and expansive.

In a human being, parts of the body are ascribed more yin or more yang qualities, as are all physiological processes and disease. To diagnose and treat back pain, for instance, a Chinese practitioner will focus on determining the yin or the yang nature of the pain as described by the patient. A yang back pain, for instance, will tend to move around, be sharp, feel tender to the touch, and respond to cold applications. A yin back pain will be more chronic and deep, achy, and tend to feel better with massage and with heat.

QI: THE LIFE FORCE

According to Chinese philosophy, all pain is caused when the yin-yang balance in the body is disturbed. Yin-yang becomes disturbed when the flow of energy through the body—energy known as "qi" (pronounced "chee")—is interrupted or blocked in some way. In Chinese medicine, qi is the energy essential for life. All of your body's functions are manifestations of qi, and your health is determined by a sufficient, balanced, and unimpeded flow of qi. Qi ensures bodily function by keeping blood and body fluids circulating to warm the body, fight disease, and protect the body against negative forces from the external environment.

Qi circulates through the body along a continuous circuit of pathways known as meridians. These meridians flow along the surface of the body and through the internal organs. When you are healthy, you have an abundance of qi flowing smoothly through the meridians and organs, which allows your body to function in balance and harmony.

If qi becomes blocked along one of your meridians, however, the organ or tissue meant to be nourished by this energy will not receive enough qi to perform its functions. By locating where in the body qi is blocked, and by releasing it through acupuncture, acupressure, herbs, and exercises, Chinese therapists attempt to restore proper energy flow to the body.

CHINESE MEDICINE AND BACK PAIN

When it comes to back pain, Chinese medicine holds that the back is governed by the channel of energy called the *bladder meridian* or the *tai yang* (bladder/small intestine) *channel*. This meridian is paired with the bladder is the *kidney meridian,* which is intimately connected with the lower back. Finally, a reservoir of protective energy, called the *governing vessel,* runs along the spine, protecting the spine and back.

As discussed in relation to Diana's case of back pain, the kidney and bladder meridians are concerned with the reserves of energy and ability that allow us to cope with stressful, busy times. Thus someone like Diana who has been under a lot of acute or chronic stress (from illness, life situations, or emotional states) will deplete these reserves. The result will be pain and/or achiness along the bladder channel (the upper and lower back) or the kidney channel (the lower back). Other symptoms, such as frequent urination, low blood sugar, fatigue at the end of the afternoon, and anxiety or fear, are all connected to this inability to hold reserves of energy, courage, and balance.

Diagnosis and Treatment of Back Pain

Like most other branches of natural medicine, Chinese medicine provides no standard diagnostic signs or treatment plans. Instead, you'll be evaluated based on your own unique constitution and energy level. Essentially, Chinese doctors attempt to treat all symptoms of disease by restoring yin-yang and a healthy qi flow to the body.

Like Diana, you might find a visit to a Chinese medical office a bit exotic. You may pick up the slightly sweet smell of burning moxa, the herb frequently used as part of acupuncture. You also might be surprised by the course the appointment takes. First, far more time than usual is spent discussing the symptoms that brought you to visit in the first place. The practitioner will ask you to be very specific about your back pain, asking you when it occurs, what it feels like (hot or cold, sharp or dull), and what makes it better.

You may also be asked more general questions about how you react to heat or cold, dampness and dryness, seasonal variations, and day to night changes in mood and feelings of well-being. Other questions might concern bowel movements, menstruation, and eating and drinking habits. Your answers to these questions will give the doctor an idea of what part of your system might be affecting your back pain and what kind of treatment you might require to bring your body back into harmony.

The physical examination that follows may also be a bit different from what you might be used to. A Chinese healer places a great deal of importance on listening to your pulse. In fact, he or she will feel twelve different pulses, six on each side, and each related to a different organ in the body. The pulses also relate to meridians, the energy pathways through the body, which may result in disease or pain if blocked.

Your Chinese doctor may also spend time looking at your tongue, just as Diana's did. According to the tenets of Chinese medicine, the tongue's coating, color, and shape reveal much about your body. By examining your tongue, the doctor is also attempting to locate where in your body qi flow has been disrupted.

Because you've come to the doctor with back pain, the practitioner will examine the energy channels that run up and down the back, legs, neck, and arms. Areas along these channels may be tender or feel warm or cool to the practiced hands of the Chinese doctor.

The bladder channel—the one most frequently affected in back problems—runs from the outside of each foot up the rear of the leg, the buttock, across the back next to the spine, up the back of the neck, and over the top of the head to end at the inside of the eye. The gallbladder channel, another likely to be affected, ascends the side of each leg, through the hip and lateral chest, across the top of the shoulder (where many of us hold our tension), and across the scalp, ending on the temple.

Once the doctor has determined the yin-yang and qi imbalance in your body, together you will plan treatment, which may include acupuncture and massage (also known as acupressure), herbal remedies, and/or qi-gong exercises. Let's take them one by one.

ACUPUNCTURE, ACUPRESSURE, AND SHIATSU

There are over one thousand "acupoints" located throughout the body. These points can be stimulated with needles or with one's own hands to enhance the flow of qi through the body and thus restore health. The points most likely to be involved in back pain are located along the bladder, gallbladder, or kidney channels. Your Chinese doctor will show you, on a chart and on your body, exactly where along these channels your difficulty is located.

Acupuncture needles are very long and very thin. Their insertion should be nearly painless, although there is often a mild pinprick and tingling sensation as the skin is pierced. Often, moxibustion is used to warm and tone the body's qi before the needles are inserted. Moxas consist of special herbs derived from the mugwort plant and are gently heated either above or on a specific acupoint.

Acupuncture needles may be inserted to a depth of about a quarter to two inches or more, depending on a variety of factors, including your size and the way that the practitioner wishes to influence the flow of qi. The practitioner always takes care to avoid blood vessels and major organs. The needles are left in place for a few seconds up to an hour; the average time is about 20 minutes. The type and extent of your back pain problem will determine how often and for how long you visit your acupuncturist. The average is about once a week for several months, then once a month or so for maintenance.

Acupressure is different from acupuncture only in that it uses finger pressure rather than needle insertion to stimulate acupoints. This method is especially helpful for those people who dislike or are afraid of needles, and it has the added comfort of physical, human touch. In addition, Chinese medical theory holds that practitioners can transfer their own qi, or energy, to you through their hands, thus helping to heal you with touch.

With a little training and guidance, you can learn to stimulate acupoints yourself and perform acupressure at home on your own. The two exercises illustrated on the next page are examples of acupressure designed to relax lower back muscles while stimulating the flow of qi through the bladder and gallbladder channels.

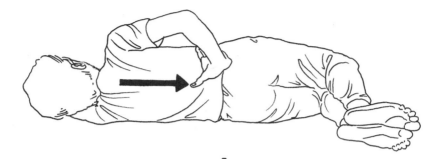

A

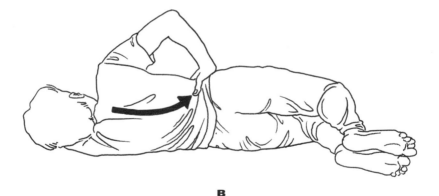

B

Do-It-Yourself Acupressure

*(a) Lie down on your side with knees bent. Using the flat part
of your thumb, stroke up and down along the spinal column from
the tailbone to as close to your shoulders as you can reach.
Repeat several times. (b) In the same position, stroke downward with
your thumb from the top of your spine and then flare outward
following the line of the ribs. Repeat this motion several times,
then turn over and repeat on opposite side.*

Shiatsu, a massage technique developed in Japan, is another method of stimulating the flow of qi. The shiatsu therapist may use a combination of fingers, thumbs, elbows, knees, and feet to press acupoints, usually in a rhythmic pattern. He or she may also stroke your body as well as gently twist your spine and other joints to further relax you.

Acupuncture, acupressure, and shiatsu all have the same goal in mind: to ensure that the life-giving energy known as qi is moving unimpeded through your body. Qi-gong exercises, described a little later in this chapter, offer another way to stimulate qi and bring your body back into balance. In addition to these methods, Chinese medicine uses herbs to nourish the body, mind, and spirit.

CHINESE HERBAL MEDICINE

The use of herbs is an essential part of traditional Chinese medicine. They are used to help reorganize the body constituents (qi, blood, and body fluids) within the meridians and the internal organs, as well as help the body to cope with stress and other external forces.

In general, Chinese herbal medicine involves using multiple herbs in combinations that have specific effects. Herbs are dispensed and can be used in many different forms, including pills, tinctures (alcohol-based solutions), or capsules. Fresh herbs may also be given, boiled in water to make teas or used in food.

The Chinese doctor you visit will suggest certain herbs for you based on your particular problem and constitution. Although it would be counterproductive to attempt to prescribe herbs for you in this text, the general principles of Chinese herbal medicine allow the practitioner to come up with an appropriate formula.

- If a pain is achy, feels better with warmth and pressure, and is deep, it is considered a cold and/or damp pain. Herbal combinations to warm it and move the dampness may include Pubescent Angelica root (*Radix Duhuo*) and Large-leaf Gentian root (*Radix Gentianae Macrophyllae*).
- If a pain is stabbing, severe, and feels warm and swollen, it is

thought of as obstruction of heat. Herbal combinations for this might include Frankincense (*Gummi Olibanum*) and Ox Knee (*Radix Achyranthis Bidentatae*).

QI-GONG: CHINESE PHYSICAL FITNESS

A third form of Chinese therapy is qi-gong, a literal translation of which is "energy exercises." Qi-gong builds qi and helps to move it freely around the body. The exercises work to cultivate inner strength, calm the mind, and help maintain the body's natural state of internal balance and harmony or, if upset, restore the balance.

There are several types of qi-gong. Some exercises are similar to calisthenic or isometric movements, others like meditative stances, still others involve the stimulation of acupressure points through massage. Breathing exercises, similar to those described in Chapter 5, are designed to bring the body into a state of relaxation and harmony.

The basic qi-gong posture involves standing with the feet apart, with knees slightly bent, back straight, and the arms held in front of the body. You are then to imagine that you are holding an imaginary "ball of qi" in front of you. This posture is maintained for a few minutes to a half hour, and will improve your circulation, warm your hands, and relax you.

Chinese medicine, with its emphasis on internal harmony and self-care, is appealing to more and more Americans every day. Anxious to avoid the often painful, usually expensive, and almost always futile mainstream treatments for back pain, millions of men and women find the ultimate goal of Chinese medicine—to bring internal harmony and balance to the body and spirit—both immediately soothing and ultimately motivating.

In Chapter 10, you'll learn about another system of medicine—one, developed in India, that also looks at health and healing from a holistic and natural perspective.

"All diseases
of the body can be
destroyed at the
root by regulating
the Prana; this is
the secret knowledge
of healing."

Swami Vishnu Devananda

Ayurveda: Medicine from India

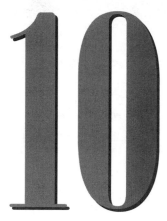

*A*fter reading about Ayurveda in a book, chronic back pain sufferer David Shepard decided to visit a yoga therapist trained in all aspects of Indian medicine. David had felt a stiffness in his lower back since college, a stiffness that seemed to have worsened in recent months. He felt very stiff in the morning, then slightly looser during the day. Even at his best, however, he found himself trying to stretch the stiffness and achiness out at every free moment.

The yoga therapist asked many questions about David's lifestyle, work habits, and diet. The practitioner asked David if he would commit to doing a series of yoga exercises every day for a month and whether he would attend a yoga class and some individual lessons during that time. David eagerly agreed to try this approach, as his visits to his regular medical doctor had resulted in plenty of x-rays and a *prescription for muscle relaxants, but no improvement in symptoms.*

The yoga exercises prescribed for David were simple and very relaxing. He was taught deep breathing and another type of breathing in which he inhaled through one nostril and exhaled out the other. Lying on his back, David learned to stretch each leg and hip, feeling the muscles of his back loosen and lengthen. The series of yoga stretches ended with the "corpse" pose, in which David stretched out on his back, making sure his lower back sank into the floor, thus relaxing his entire back and body.

David learned to begin each day by performing 20 minutes of yoga exercises. Almost immediately, he found that yoga, combined with a hot shower afterward, made his back feel looser than ever. The therapist gave him some herbs and ginger to use in a bath three to four evenings per week. David was also instructed to send away for some powdered Ayurvedic herbs, which he was told would "purify" his blood, diminishing the toxins that had built up in his system and prevented proper fluid motion in his body. The therapist also suggested some dietary changes, including eliminating "nightshade" foods like tomatoes, potatoes, and peppers, because these foods tend to increase inflammation.

After a few weeks, David's routine of yoga in the morning and periodic nighttime baths seemed like a normal, and much welcome, part of his life. He continued to take yoga classes, learned to meditate in order to reduce stress and increase his sense of inner balance, and began to work with the Ayurvedic doctor on diet and herbal treatment for his back pain as well as for other long-term problems. Physically and spiritually, he felt better than ever.

Ayurveda: Knowledge of Life

In Sanskrit, the primary language of ancient India, Ayurveda means "knowledge of life." Indeed, it is far more than a compendium of medical treatments, instead representing a complete philosophy of life and living. Like its cousin, traditional Chinese medicine, Ayurvedic medicine sees each individual as an extension of the universe, and health as a state of balance within the body and between the body and the universe. In Ayurveda, as in most holistic views of health and healing, there is no dividing line between body, mind, and spirit, and disease and pain can be caused by physical, psychological, or spiritual imbalances. Your case of back pain, for instance, could very well stem from the fact that your life is too filled with stress or that you are unhappy in your relationships with others.

Ayurvedic medicine attempts to treat not just the presenting symptoms, but the whole body. It uses a combination of herbal medicine, diet, yoga, and meditation to bring the body back into balance. And as is true in many forms of alternative medicine, the process of diagnosis in Ayurvedic medicine relies far more on a practitioner's powers of observation and questioning than on laboratory tests or imaging techniques.

THE DIAGNOSTIC TECHNIQUE

If you're like most Americans and more familiar with Western techniques, you may be surprised when the Ayurvedic practitioner begins to smell and touch your skin in examining all aspects of your body and personal behavior. Don't be alarmed, however; this is how your condition will be diagnosed and a treatment plan devised.

The Ayurvedic practitioner will probably begin your examination by taking your pulse. In fact, he or she will listen to your pulse at 12 separate sites on the wrists—6 on the left and 6 on the right. Measuring the pulses informs the practitioner of the movement of energy—called *prana*—through the body, as well as the general health of each internal organ.

Another important diagnostic tool used in Ayurvedic medicine, as well as in traditional Chinese medicine, is the examination of the tongue. In Ayurveda, the tongue is divided into areas which reflect the different organs, and the coating on the tongue reflects the amount and type of toxins in the organs. For instance, the rear of the tongue corresponds to the lower back and kidney area; thus a practitioner may look there first if you come in complaining of low-back pain.

In addition, you'll be asked a great many questions about your medical history, your present symptoms, and your general feelings about your personal life and physical condition. Not only will the practitioner take note of *what* you say, but also the *way* you say it: the strength and sincerity (or lack thereof) of your voice may reflect your willingness to accept responsibility for your own health. Based on the results of these and other examination procedures, an Ayurvedic doctor will attempt to locate your physical and emotional strengths and weaknesses, as prescribed by Ayurvedic tenets. We discuss some of those tenets in the section below, before we cover specific therapies for back pain.

The ABCs of Ayurvedic Philosophy

As you explore Ayurvedic principles in relation to your back pain, keep in mind that Ayurveda teaches that all of life—including disease and its symptoms—depends upon learning and developing self-knowledge. In this way, back pain can be seen as an opportunity to reexamine your spiritual life and physical state in order to correct any imbalances and thus bring your body back into alignment with the energy of nature and the universe. Later in this chapter, we'll show you some of the ways Ayurvedic therapies may be used to treat back pain. In the meantime, here is a brief overview of Ayurvedic philosophy.

PRANA: THE LIFE FORCE AND THE THREE DOSHAS

Known as *qi* in Chinese medicine, the life-providing energy in Ayurveda is called *prana*. Prana is the animating power of life, providing vitality and endurance to each human being. Prana is also considered to be the power behind the healing process. Indeed, Ayurveda teaches that we each have a Divine Healer within us that, if properly directed, can restore health and balance to the body.

Balance is a particularly important theme in Ayurvedic medicine, as it is in traditional Chinese medicine. In this Indian philosophy, balance and harmony are maintained by what are known as the *three doshas,* forces of energy that act upon body substances and organs. When the three doshas are balanced, the body functions harmoniously and in health; when they are out of balance, disease results.

The three doshas are called *vata, pitta,* and *kapha.* Vata represents movement; pitta, metabolism and heat; and kapha, structure. Within every cell of the body, these three operating principles must exist in proper balance for health to be maintained. A balance between the doshas will allow your physical, emotional, and intellectual qualities to function with vitality and energy.

According to Ayurvedic tenets, each individual has a specific body type based on one of the three doshas. In essence, one of these qualities—movement, heat, or stability—predominates, helping to form your unique personality and physiology. Your Ayurvedic body type is like a blueprint outlining the innate tendencies that have been built into your system. It helps to explain why you are able to consume lots of salt without suffering any ill effects, while your sister's blood pressure soars when she overloads on sodium. Or why nightshade foods like eggplant cause a flare-up of your back pain, but have no adverse consequences for your sister. Since a prime goal of Ayurvedic medicine is to prevent disease from occurring in the first place, understanding one's own dosha and practicing a lifestyle designed to maintain dosha balance is essential. Furthermore, by accurately identifying your body type, an Ayurvedic practitioner then is able to diagnose and treat your condition more effectively.

Your dosha is determined by your body shape, your personality, and many other physical and emotional attributes. Below are short descriptions of each type of dosha as it applies to body type:

Vata, pronounced (vah-tah), represents the force of movement within your body. It activates the physical system and is responsible for respiration and blood flow through the body. The seats of vata—the places in the body from which it springs—are the large intestine, pelvic cavity, skin, ears, and thighs. Organs associated with vata include the bone, the brain (especially motor activity), the heart, and the lungs.

If you are predominantly a vata body type, you tend to be rather thin, with prominent features, and cool, dry skin. You're inclined to speak rapidly and have an active, creative mind. You probably like to keep irregular hours, and may be prone to feel anxious and worried. Vata's season is autumn—a dry, windy season during which vata people often develop arthritis, rheumatism, constipation, and other diseases of the vata organs.

The *pitta* dosha governs the metabolic processes of cells. Organs associated with pitta include the blood, the brain (especially memory and learning), hormones, liver, small intestine, and spleen. If you're a pitta body type, you tend to have a medium build, thin hair, and warm, ruddy skin. Pittas are organized, work hard, and have very regular sleeping and eating patterns. Although generally warm and loving, a person with a predominantly pitta dosha may also display quick bursts of temper. Pittas tend to suffer from acne, hemorrhoids, and ulcers, and may often feel warm and thirsty. The pitta season is summer, when the heat and bright light may aggravate pitta-related disorders, including rashes, diarrhea, and inflammatory conditions.

Finally, *kapha* dosha is responsible for physical strength and stability. It holds together the structure of the body and is located in the chest, lungs, and spinal fluid. Organs associated with kapha include the brain (information storage), joints, lymph, and stomach. If you have a predominantly kapha body type, you tend to be heavyset, with cool, oily skin. Kaphas are often very relaxed and tolerant people, who are slow to anger and have a tendency to procrastinate. They sleep for long hours and may not eat for the physical reasons but rather for the emotional pleasure that food brings to them. Kapha types are especially prone to obesity as well as to illnesses of the kapha organs, such as allergies and sinus problems. The kapha season is winter, when the respiratory system is particularly susceptible to colds and congestion.

Ayurveda and Back Pain

According to Ayurvedic philosophy, most cases of lower-back pain stem from an imbalance of *apana vata,* the "subdosha" of vata that controls the lower back and intestinal tract. Vata is connected with the nervous system, specifically the impulses traveling along nerves, muscles, and blood vessels wherever there is movement in the body. Located in the colon and lower abdomen, the apana vata is responsible for muscle movement in the lower back and the elimination of wastes from the digestive tract, as well as sexual function and menstruation. Thus relieving lower-back pain generally involves bringing apana vata back into balance.

THE AYURVEDIC PRESCRIPTION

All treatment for back pain—indeed, for all illnesses—involves the use of diet and nutrition, herbs, yoga exercises, meditation, massage, and breathing exercises. It is important to remember that Ayurvedic medicine does not treat any condition in isolation, and thus the whole body must be brought into balance before a specific symptom, like back pain, can be alleviated.

The first step in your treatment may involve what is called *panchakarma,* which is the process of detoxifying your body of impurities or toxins. Detoxification may consist of induced vomiting, enemas, blood cleansing (by blood-letting and using blood-thinning herbs), and nasal douching—all under the strict and careful supervision of the Ayurvedic practitioner. Yoga, chanting, meditation, and lying in the sun for long periods make up another stage in the cleansing process.

A period of *tonification,* or enhancement, then takes place. During tonification, you'll consume certain herbs and perform particular yoga and breathing exercises. At the same time, or perhaps as a next stage in the healing process, you'll spend a great deal of time meditating; this is called *satvajaya* and has as its goal the reduction of psychological and emotional stress, as well as the release of negative emotions and ideas.

Although the foregoing steps are recommended for anyone desiring to attain proper health and balance, those who suffer from back pain are likely to be prescribed certain specific dietary guidelines, herbal remedies, and yoga exercises designed to bring their apana vata back into balance. These prescriptions tend to be quite personal and individual in nature; everyone with lower-back pain does not have the same physical makeup and thus will not respond to the same treatments.

Eating Plan. Dietary measures are particularly personal. Based on your own specific needs and physiology, the Ayurvedic practitioner will devise an eating plan that is designed to help restore your health and alleviate your back pain. In most cases, a diet to pacify or moderate the apana vata subdosha would include increasing the amount of asparagus, cooked onions, garlic, and okra, while avoiding broccoli, cabbage, eggplant and other vegetables of the nightshade family like potatoes and mushrooms. Dried fruits, beans, and certain herbs, like coriander seed and saffron, are among the other foods that an Ayurvedic prescription for back pain might limit or eliminate from the diet. However, you should work closely with your practitioner to devise an eating plan that works for you.

Herbal Supplements. There are more than 2,000 different herbs that are used as drugs in mainstream as well as Ayurvedic and Chinese medicine. Among those used most often to treat back pain are the following:

- Fo-ti (*Polygonum multiflorem*): This root herb, also used in Chinese medicine, is thought to help strengthen muscles, tendons, ligaments, and bones. It is most often taken as a tea made by steeping one-half ounce of the root in one pint of water. Fo-ti is often used to treat back pain in combination with another herb, called gotu kola.
- Gotu kola (*Hydrocotyle asiatica*): This is the essential revitalizing herb for the nerves and brain cells. It is a tonic and rejuvenative for pitta. At the same time, it inhibits vata, calming the nerves, and helps reduce excess kapha, which can exacerbate inflammation.
- Rehmannia (*Rehmannia glutinosa*): Another root also used in Chinese medicine, rehmannia is kapha in nature, thereby increasing bodily tissues, secretions, and fluids. It is particularly helpful in flushing out the digestive system, which may alleviate back pain caused or exacerbated by constipation. It is available in powder form, which can be used to make tea.

Yoga. Yoga exercises are meant to stimulate and stretch your muscles and organs, as well as bring your mind and body into a deeper state of relaxation. There are dozens of yoga techniques and exercises and, in fact, several different schools of yoga, each one with a slightly different philosophy and emphasis. Indeed, the study of yoga in its fullest measure and many levels is a lifetime endeavor, one that Ayurvedic tradition dictates leads to true harmony and health.

At the same time, however, yoga poses in and of themselves can be quite helpful in alleviating back pain. Yoga poses, performed correctly and practiced regularly, will help you keep your body in balance and the muscles and tendons of your back supple and lithe.

In particular, three yoga poses are especially useful for back pain problems:

- *Cobra pose:* This pose helps to strengthen the back and stretch the abdominal muscles.
    1. Start by lying face down on your stomach. Bring your feet together and place your hands directly under your shoulders, fingers pointing forward.
    2. Breathe in deeply, expanding your chest forward. As you do so, press down with your hands and lift the chest off the floor slowly until your arms are fully extended. Be sure to keep your elbows close to your sides and your shoulders down away from your ears.
    3. Hold this pose, then slowly release while exhaling. Repeat the pose three times.
- *Locust pose:* Another pose designed to strengthen the lower back, the locust pose also aids in digestion and the process of urination.
    1. Lie face down with your chin resting gently on the floor. Place your arms back by your sides, next to your hips, or under your thighs, palms pointing toward the ceiling.
    2. Inhale deeply, raising both legs at the same time by stretching out from the hips. Feel your spine lengthen as your legs extend upward and back. Keep breathing, slowly and regularly, while holding this pose for 5 to 10 seconds.
    3. Release the legs slowly, then repeat the pose three times.

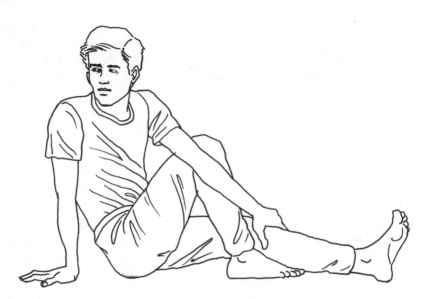

Simple Yoga Posture

*Sit on the floor with your legs straight out in front
of you. Bend your left knee and place your left hand on the floor
slightly behind you. Hold your right leg just below the knee,
placing your right elbow on the outside of your bent left leg.*

*Take a deep breath and, as you do so, lift your rib
cage and lengthen your spine upward. As you exhale, twist from
the base of your spine to the left. Let your head follow the
movement of your spine. Keep breathing while you hold the pose
for several seconds. Release slowly and return to the
starting position. Repeat to the other side.*

- *Seated twisted pose:* In addition to soothing and calming the mind and toning the internal organs, this pose helps to stretch the spine and bring blood and nutrients to the back muscles.
  1. Sit up straight, with your legs extended in front of you.
  2. Bend your left knee, placing the sole of your left foot flat on the floor as close to your right knee or thigh as possible. Extend your right leg as much as possible to lengthen your spine.
  3. Place your left hand on the floor behind you, while bringing your right arm to the outside of the left knee. If you are flexible, your right elbow should be flush with the outside of your left knee. If you are a beginner, you can simply grasp your knee with your right hand.
  4. Inhale deeply, opening up the chest while bringing it to the left. Let your head follow the movement of your spine as it twists. Twist as far as you can without straining your muscles.
  5. Keep breathing normally while holding this pose for 10 to 15 seconds, then release slowly.
  6. Repeat the pose two more times on this side, then reverse your position, twisting to the right three times.

Now that you've received an overview of Ayurvedic techniques and traditions, we hope you'll take the time to further explore this complex system of healing in more depth (see *Natural Resources*, page 188, for more information). In the meantime, let's take a look at another form of alternative medicine that uses the power of herbs and aromas to help restore and maintain health.

"Speak to the earth, and it shall teach thee."

Job 12:8

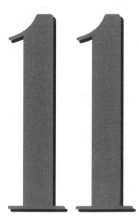

The Healing Power of Herbs and Aromas

$\mathcal{S}$ometime between 1000 and 700 B.C., a Chinese emperor named Shen Nung compiled a list of some 350 plants known to have medicinal value. Called the *Pen Tsao,* or *Great Herbal,* this text represents the earliest written herbal handbook. In every culture throughout history, humanity has depended on the nutritional value and healing power of flowers, herbs, barks, heartwoods, ferns, mosses, lichens, seaweed, and fungi. Herbal remedies form an important part of many types of traditional approaches to medicine and health, including Chinese medicine and Ayurveda. Although these systems share a common goal—the restoration of internal harmony—each may use herbs in a slightly different way, depending upon how the body is viewed and the condition diagnosed. Even modern mainstream medicine is intimately linked to herbal medicine: Approximately 25 percent of all prescription drugs in the United States are derived from trees, shrubs, or herbs. Many other drugs are synthesized to mimic a natural plant compound.

A close relative of herbal medicine is a branch of natural medicine known as aromatherapy. Dating back to ancient Egypt in about 4500 B.C., aromatherapy is a method of treating illness through the inhalation and external application of essential oils derived from the roots, stems, seeds, and flowers of plants.

A visit to an herbalist is highly recommended for anyone who suffers from either an acute back injury or chronic back pain. Like other alternative therapies, herbal medicine attempts not to cure disease per se, but rather to help the body remain in, or return itself to, the state of balance we know of as health. In this attempt, herbalists explore lifestyle and dietary habits with their patients to develop an individualized treatment plan. This exploration generally goes far beyond what one would experience with most mainstream physicians.

Although each person who visits an herbalist is likely to emerge with a different prescription (even for the very same complaint), there are some generalities that can be made about possible remedies. There are antispasmodic agents to ease cramps in smooth and skeletal muscles; anti-inflammatories to soothe inflammations or reduce the inflammatory response related to sprains and strains; and nervines and tonics that strengthen and restore the nervous system, helping to relieve tension and stress. A variety of essential oils are used for generally the same purposes: to soothe aching muscles and to help relax the body and mind.

During your first appointment with an herbalist, you should expect the practitioner to take a complete medical history which concentrates on the exact nature of your back pain, the level and type of your physical activity, and any past medical and surgical treatments for back pain you may have received. If the herbalist is a medical doctor or other trained professional, he or she may also perform a physical exam. It is highly likely that the herbalist would recommend that you visit a chiropractor or osteopath for treatment as well. (See Chapter 8 for more information on these forms of treatment.) Based on what is discovered during the exam, the herbalist would then prescribe one or more natural medications aimed at strengthening your constitution while alleviating your symptoms.

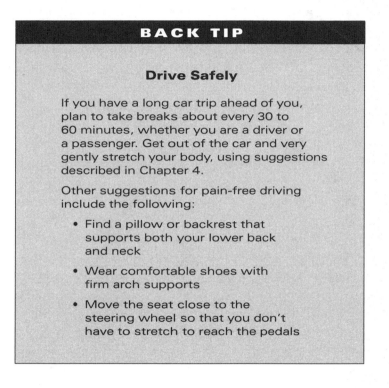

BACK TIP

Drive Safely

If you have a long car trip ahead of you, plan to take breaks about every 30 to 60 minutes, whether you are a driver or a passenger. Get out of the car and very gently stretch your body, using suggestions described in Chapter 4.

Other suggestions for pain-free driving include the following:

- Find a pillow or backrest that supports both your lower back and neck

- Wear comfortable shoes with firm arch supports

- Move the seat close to the steering wheel so that you don't have to stretch to reach the pedals

Herbal Medicine: Nature's Pharmacy

In general, herbal medicines work in much the same way as conventional pharmaceutical drugs. Herbs contain a large number of naturally occurring substances that work to alter the body's chemistry in order to return it to its natural state of health. Unlike purified drugs, however, plants contain a wide variety of substances and, hence, less of any one particular active chemical. This attribute makes plants far less toxic to the body than most pharmaceutical products.

Another benefit of natural herbs is that they tend to contain combinations of substances that work together to restore balance to the
body with a minimum of side effects. An example is the plant meadowsweet, which contains anti-inflammatory compounds similar to the
ones in aspirin used to treat back pain and other musculoskeletal ailments. These compounds, called salicylates, often irritate the stomach
lining. Unlike commercially prepared aspirin, however, meadowsweet
also contains substances that soothe the gastric lining and reduce
stomach acidity, thus providing relief from pain while protecting the
stomach from irritation. For people with chronic back pain who have
been forced to choose between backaches and stomachaches, such a
treatment can seem like an absolute godsend.

Herbs of all types are available in many forms including:

- *Whole herbs:* Plants or plant parts that are dried and either cut
  or powdered to be used as teas or as cooking herbs.
- *Capsules and tablets:* A fast-growing corner of the herbal medicine market consists of capsules and tablets, which allow
  herbs to be taken quickly and without requiring the individual
  to taste them.
- *Extracts and tinctures:* Extracts and tinctures are made by grind-
  ing the roots, leaves, and/or flowers of an herb and immersing
  them in a solution of alcohol and water for a period of time. The
  alcohol works both to extract the maximum amount of active
  ingredients from the herb and to act as a preservative.

HERBS TO TREAT BACK PAIN

Here are the herbs most likely to be recommended for back pain:

Black Cohosh (*Cimicifuga racemosa*). A remedy first used by
North American Indians, this herb acts as a muscle relaxant and is useful in treating pain related to osteoarthritis, sciatica, and back spasm.

Preparation and dosage: Black cohosh is administered as a
tea, which can be made by steeping ½ to 1 teaspoon of the dried herb
in a cup of boiling water for about 10 minutes. Drink the tea three
times a day.

Cramp Bark (*Viburnum opulus*). As its name suggests, this herb derived from the bark of a tree works to relieve muscle spasms and cramping and thus is quite helpful to anyone in the acute phase of back pain.

Preparation and dosage: To make a tea, put 2 teaspoons of dried bark into a cup of water, bring to a boil, then simmer for 15 minutes. Drink a cup three times a day. Use 4 to 8 drops of the tincture three times a day.

Horse Chestnut (*Aesculus hippocastanum*). Prepared from chestnuts gathered as they fall ripe from trees in autumn, this remedy works as a tonic for the circulatory system, thus reducing the inflammatory response in the strained muscles of the back.

Preparation and dosage: Horse chestnut is available as a tea or as an ointment. Tea is prepared by pouring a cup of boiling water onto 1 or 2 teaspoons of dried chestnut and allowing the herb to steep for 15 to 20 minutes. The liquid can then be either drunk (three times a day) or used as a lotion. Ointment dosage is 1 to 4 drops three times a day.

Willow Bark (*Salix nigra*). The bark of this willow tree is a natural source of the aspirinlike salicylates. It acts as an antiinflammatory and analgesic.

Preparation and dosage: Willow bark can be drunk as a tea (steep 2 teaspoons of bark in a cup of boiling water for 10 minutes) or applied as an ointment (2 to 4 ml) three times a day.

The Healing Power of Scent

The term *aromatherapy* was coined in 1937 by the French chemist René-Maurice Gattefossé, who badly burned his hand during a laboratory experiment in his family's perfume factory. Knowing that lavender was used in medicine for burns, he plunged his hand into a vat of pure lavender oil used to make perfume. After noticing that his hand healed very quickly, Gattefossé began to explore the healing powers of other essential oils.

Essential oils, composed of the plant's most volatile constituents, are extracted from plants through a process of steam distillation or cold pressing. To derive pure essential oils, no other chemicals or substances should be used during the extraction process since they would disrupt the natural organic composition of plant material. Indeed, each essential oil is made up of several different organic molecules that, working together, give the oil its unique perfume as well as its particular therapeutic qualities.

Like the plants and herbs from which they are extracted, some essential oils are known to have antiviral and antibacterial properties and thus can be used to treat infections such as herpes simplex, skin and bowel infections, and the flu. Perhaps the most commonly used aromatherapy is one that uses oil derived from the eucalyptus plant which, when inhaled, works to restore health to the respiratory system by acting as an antibacterial, antiviral agent as well as an expectorant.

Other therapeutic oils ease the antiinflammatory response in the body, making them especially useful in treating back pain as well as arthritis and similar conditions. In addition, there are a number of oils that have profound effects on the nervous system. Stress, as you may remember from Chapter 5, overstimulates the sympathetic nervous system and forces the muscles to tense up and, eventually, to shorten. Certain essential oils, when inhaled, can help to bring the sympathetic nervous system into balance with the actions of the parasympathetic nervous system and thus reduce the negative effects stress may have on the musculoskeletal system.

USING AROMATHERAPY

Essential oils are delicate, highly concentrated essences of plants. The quantity of plant material needed to make even a small amount of essential oil is enormous: To make an ounce of lavender oil, for instance, requires about 12 pounds of fresh lavender flowers. Fortunately, only a very small amount of oil is needed to have therapeutic effects.

You can buy essential oils in their pure form or already diluted with another base oil, usually made from olives, soy, or almonds. In addition, herbs that "fix" the scents are added, so that the potency of the mixture is maintained over time. Combining essences with base oils does not change their chemical composition, but will help to reduce their potential toxicity to the skin or internal tissue.

Although it is possible to make your own essential oils with a homemade still, most people choose to purchase prepared oils from health-food stores and/or mail-order companies. However, it is important that you make sure that the essential oils you use are just that: essential, meaning that their original chemical compositions were not altered in any way during the extraction process. Make sure that when you buy oils the word "essential" is used on the label and that you buy your oils from a reputable dealer. (See *Natural Resources*, page 188, for more information on obtaining essential oils.)

In general, there are two main ways to use essential oils:

As Inhalants. Simply breathing in the odors and minute particles of plant material will help bring your body back into balance. There are several equally effective methods of inhaling essential oils:

- *Aroma lamps:* Putting a few drops of oil on a light bulb or burning a candle under a cup that has drops of oil in it will volatize the oil into the atmosphere, making your whole environment rich with soothing aroma.
- *Diffusors:* Mechanical devices disperse microparticles of essential oils into the air.
- *Facial saunas:* Pour boiling water into a bowl, then add a few drops of essential oil. Drape a towel over your head and lean over the bowl so that the towel encloses both head and bowl. The essences are thus absorbed both through the skin and through the membranes of the nasal passages.

As Topical Applications. When diluted properly with base oils, essential oils may be safely and effectively applied directly to the skin. (If any essential oil seems to irritate your skin, however, discontinue use.)

- *Bath oils:* Adding a few drops of an essential oil to bathwater both adds to the relaxing atmosphere and allows the oils to seep into the skin. Warm baths are also helpful in easing sore, strained back muscles.
- *Massage:* Oils can be massaged into the face, back, chest, or any other part of the body that is feeling pain or stress. A tiny bit of essential oil gently rubbed into the temples each evening can melt away the day's tension. As mentioned in Chapter 7, massage itself, especially when performed by someone trained in the art, is an integral part of any treatment for chronic back pain as it both releases tension and helps the muscles and joints move back into alignment.
- *Poultice:* An age-old way of relieving chronic pain and stiffness, poultices are made by moistening raw herbs and applying them directly to the affected area.

AROMATHERAPY AND BACK PAIN

The following is a list of essential oils that may help to ease your back pain, either by reducing inflammation or by relieving the stress and tension that trigger and aggravate the pain. Please note that this is a highly subjective list and that many other oils may work just as well, if not better, depending on your own individual constitution and needs. That's why it is important that you visit an herbalist trained in aromatherapy to learn more about how to apply this ancient art to your particular health problem.

Aspic (*Lavandula spica*). Cultivated in Spain from a variety of lavender, the aspic plant exudes an oil that can be massaged into aching muscles. In fact, European veterinarians often rub aspic oil into the backs and legs of racehorses to soothe their muscles after a race. Aspic oil is also known as an excellent topical remedy for skin irritations like acne, excema, and burns.

Clary Sage/Sage Oil (*Salvia officinalis*). Distilled from the flowering tops and leaves of a common perennial plant, clary sage oil has long been known for its medicinal properties. Clary sage oil is an all-around tonic that can help reduce fatigue, irritability, and depression and thus help to bolster self-esteem and reduce overall stress on the body.

Frankincense Oil (*Boswellia carteri*). Frankincense has been used since ancient times in religious ritual and remains today a major ingredient of church incense, no doubt because of its ability to help individuals who breathe its scent to attain a deeper state of meditation and prayer. For that reason, it is recommended for people with stress-related back pain.

Juniper (*Juniperus communis*). Steam-distilled from the crushed dried fruit of the juniper berry, juniper oil is often used as an antiseptic as well as a diuretic. When mixed with wheat germ or olive oil, it can be massaged into any stiff joint—including those at the back of the neck and in the lumbar spine—to relieve inflammation.

Lavender (*Lavandula angustifolia*). The classic oil of aromatherapy, lavender has a wide range of therapeutic qualities. Used topically, it can help heal burns, wounds, and insect bites. For patients with stress-related back pain, it can work to bring the body back into harmony by calming the sympathetic nervous system and stimulating the parasympathetic nervous system.

Mandarin (*Citrus reticulata*). Derived from the peel of the mandarin orange, this essential oil is a soothing and calming potion when used as a massage oil or in a warm bath. People who have trouble sleeping may find its soothing effects especially helpful at bedtime.

Neroli (*Citrus aurantium bigaradia*). Neroli oil is obtained by the steam distillation of the flowers of the Seville orange, native to the Mediterranean region. It is known as an effective antispasmodic and a great stress reliever—a perfect combination for anyone with chronic back pain.

Rosemary (*Rosmarinus officinalis*). One of the best-known and most often used aromatic herbs, rosemary oil is steam-distilled from the tops, leaves, and smaller twigs of the plant. It has been used for centuries to treat a variety of conditions, including stomach and liver problems, infections of all kinds, and depression. Used in a poultice, as a massage oil, or in the bath, rosemary is a muscle relaxant and a stress reducer.

Keep in mind that, as is true of all forms of natural medicine, aromatherapy is highly individualized. An oil that relaxes one individual may work to stimulate another. Therefore, you may want to experiment by using a few different oils, alone or in combination, until you find a regimen that works best for your needs. In addition, remember always that essential oils are, in fact, potent drugs and should thus be used with care.

Here are some other tips about aromatherapy:

- Before you use any essential oil on your skin, whether in the bath, as a liniment, or as a massage oil, make sure you first perform a patch test. To do so, wash about a two-inch-square area on your forearm and dry it carefully. Apply a tiny drop of the essential oil, diluting it with an equal part of a bland oil, like olive oil. Then place a Band-Aid over the area and wait 24 hours. If no irritation occurs, use the oil in your formulas. If you have a reaction—such as a rash or blisters—look for another oil. A patch test is especially important if you have allergies or particularly sensitive skin.
- If you are pregnant, check with both your obstetrician and your alternative practitioner before using any essential oils.
- Do not take essential oils internally unless you first discuss the matter thoroughly with your practitioner.
- Keep essential oils out of your eyes.
- Store essential oils in dark glass or metal bottles and protect them from light and heat.

Herbal medicine and its cousin aromatherapy are two of the fastest-growing branches of alternative medicine in the United States. Please see *Natural Resources*, page 188, to locate organizations that can provide you with more information as well as discover the titles to some helpful books about aromatherapy and herbal medicine. In the next chapter, we'll explore another branch of natural therapy called homeopathy.

"The natural healing force within each one of us is the greatest force in getting well."

Hippocrates

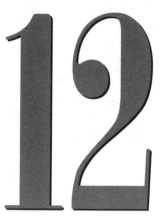

Homeopathy
and Back Pain

*D*erived from the Greek work *homoios* (meaning "similar") and *pathos* (meaning "suffering"), homeopathy was developed by nineteenth-century German physician Samuel Hahnemann. Homeopathy represents a striking alternative to the way modern medicine looks at health and disease, particularly chronic conditions such as most cases of back pain.

As we've seen with many of the alternative therapies discussed in this book, however, it is impossible to describe how a homeopath would diagnose or treat your particular case of back pain. Your prescription would be based completely on your own unique symptoms, lifestyle, and personal needs. In fact, like other practitioners of alternative medicine, a homeopath may not consider the source of back pain to be a muscle strain, or a herniated lumbar disc, or sciatica, or even excess stress, but instead locate the source of the problem else-where in the body or mind.

Samuel Hahnemann was a deeply spiritual man who believed that a physician's role should be to help a patient's own body heal itself, that true healing could not take place by simply administering drugs that would, in essence, override the body's natural processes. Inside every human, Hahnemann believed, was a "vital force," a life power that animates and rules the body, keeping it in balance and health. Disease occurs when a disturbance of this vital force takes place. Homeopathy considers symptoms of disease to be the external evi-dence of the vital force's internal attempts to bring the body back to a state of balance. An aching back, for instance, might represent the body's effort to correct a spinal misalignment or release accumulated toxins and waste products from the muscles.

To help the body in its own efforts to heal itself—to strengthen its vital force against an illness—a homeopath administers remedies designed to match the symptoms, not to alleviate them as Western med-icine is designed to do. This principle is known as Hahnemann's *law of similars,* or "like cures like." By making symptoms temporarily worse, a remedy would be strengthening the body's own power to heal itself. In fact, in the view of homeopathy, any therapy that attempts to sup-press the free flow of symptoms will actually prolong the underlying disturbance, since it prevents the body from being able to heal itself.

Another theory of homeopathic medicine is known as the *law of infinitesimals.* First developed by Hahnemann in order to reduce the side effects of often potentially toxic chemicals, this theory states that the smaller the dose of medicine, the greater its potency and its effect on the body's vital force. Homeopathic remedies are extracts derived by soaking plant, animal, or mineral substances in alcohol to form what is known as the "mother tincture." This tincture is again diluted with alcohol in ratios of 1 part tincture to 10 or 100 parts of alcohol, shaken vigorously, then diluted again.

This process of shaking and diluting, repeated several times, is known as "succussion." Many researchers believe that through suc-cussion the vital energy of a substance is transferred to the tincture.

Therefore, the more times the solution is passed through succussion, the more potent the remedy, even though there appears to be no trace of the original herb or mineral left. Finally, the resulting solution is added to tablets, usually made of sugar.

Prescriptions for homeopathic remedies are written only after a homeopath carefully evaluates a patient's particular set of symptoms and physical and emotional make-up. Indeed, a session with a homeopath may be a unique experience for those of us who are accustomed to Western medicine's approach to diagnosis and treatment. A homeopath will spend much more time talking to a patient about symptoms and lifestyle factors, and looking more carefully at demeanor, personality, and coloring, than a mainstream physician.

According to homeopathic tenets, mental and emotional disturbances are more serious than physical illnesses, primarily because they can themselves cause physical disease. Back pain is a perfect example. High stress levels and the emotions they provoke (such as anger, anxiety, and irritability) are directly linked to muscle spasms and strains that are at the heart of most cases of back pain. A homeopath will spend a great deal of time talking to you about stress and your ability to cope with it before he or she makes a diagnosis or prescribes a remedy.

In fact, the way a homeopath treats diseases or conditions like back pain depends entirely on an individual's particular pattern of symptoms. Not everyone with lower-back pain, for instance, can trace the problem to a herniated disc or even to general stress and tension. Nor does the pain occur at the same time or in the same place or for the same reasons in every patient. A conventional, mainstream physician will offer the same treatment—or lack of treatment in the case of many people with chronic pain—to almost everyone. Usually this consists of a combination of painkillers, exercise, and/or surgery. A homeopath, on the other hand, recognizes several different symptom patterns and has corresponding remedies for each one. The symptoms of the patient are matched with the pattern of symptoms produced by a remedy. The more closely the remedy matches the total symptom pattern of the patient, the more effective the remedy will be.

Furthermore, the symptoms that first bring a patient to the doctor (called *common symptoms* in homeopathy) are rarely the most important symptoms when it comes to selecting a remedy. Instead, *general symptoms,* which include the patient's state of mind and mood, are given more weight in determining a treatment. Other symptoms, called *particular symptoms,* are those that pertain to any given organ or structure of the body (muscle pain, for instance). They, too, are less important than the general symptoms. Most important of all are what homeopaths call *strange, rare, and peculiar symptoms*; as their name implies, they are symptoms that are completely unique to the individual patient describing them. A man who says that his back feels like it is on fire and a woman who feels as if she is trapped inside her skin are examples of two people with strange, rare, and peculiar symptoms. Even if each of them also experiences lower-back pain, each would probably be given a different remedy.

In addition, an important aspect of homeopathy is the *law of cure,* which postulates that symptoms disappear in the reverse order of appearance. In other words, the last symptoms to appear will be the first to disappear with treatment. If a patient has had many health problems through the years, he or she may find symptoms of past problems reappearing as homeopathic treatment continues. Someone who comes to a homeopath for back pain, for instance, may find that symptoms of bronchitis, a previous illness, briefly develop. Slowly but surely, working backward in time, the homeopathic remedy or remedies will restore strength to the vital force and balance to the internal environment.

Treating Back Pain with Homeopathy

Because treatment is dependent on symptoms, any of the several hundred homeopathic remedies described in Hahnemann's *Materia Medica Pura,* upon which modern homeopathy is based, might be prescribed for a person with back pain. In addition, a homeopath would work with an individual to resolve the underlying physical and emotional problems that contribute to the pain. A sculptor who spends his day bending over a table full of clay is unlikely to find a permanent solution to his lower backache in any bottle or tablet—at least not until he corrects his postural imbalances by either strengthening his abdominal and back muscles or changing the height of his table, or both.

That said, there are some general recommendations for homeopathic remedies that might apply to you. Among them are the following:

Arnica montana: So named because it grows in the mountains of Europe and the northwestern United States, this herb is one of the most often used in homeopathy. It is effective for treating a wide range of conditions, including heart disease, cuts and scrapes, and gastrointestinal disorders as well as back pain. Used topically as a tincture or ointment, arnica can soothe muscles that are aching and sore from an acute injury or from chronic misuse. The patient for whom *Arnica montana* might be prescribed complains of feeling bruised and cold, and tends to have nightmares.

Pulsatilla: This perennial herb, also known as meadow anemone, is a remedy often used to treat symptoms of premenstrual syndrome, but is also useful in treating pains in the extremities and the spine. The individual for whom *Pulsatilla* might work best is someone who seems eager to please, highly emotional, and affectionate. Symptoms tend to worsen when he or she is in a warm room but improve in open air.

Rhus toxicodendron: Believe it or not, one of the most effective homeopathic remedies for inflammation associated with back strain is derived from the poison ivy plant. *Rhus tox.,* as it is often abbreviated, was first used as a medicine in 1798. This substance affects the skin and mucous membranes, as well as joints, tendons, and muscles. *Rhus tox.* relieves immediate symptoms of soreness when rubbed into the affected area and can also act to prevent further damage after an acute injury. The individual for whom *Rhus tox.* is appropriate complains that symptoms tend to be worse at the beginning of a movement and improve with activity. He or she tends to be restless, have trouble sleeping, and suffer frequent headaches.

The treatment of any disorder with homeopathy, including back pain and other musculoskeletal disorders, requires ongoing observation and, in some cases, a series of different remedies prescribed on the basis of new, emerging symptoms. Fortunately, the remedies tend to be relatively inexpensive. And once a person's condition and makeup are well-understood by both the homeopath and the patient him- or herself, the remedies may be self-administered at home.

When German physician Samuel Hahnemann first developed homeopathy, modern medicine was in its infancy. The emerging modern pharmacy and operating room were on their way to becoming the mainstays of Western medicine. The World Health Organization estimates that some 500 million people around the world now use homeopathy as a treatment for disease even as high-tech medicine continues to dominate the scene. If you are interested in exploring homeopathy as a treatment option for your back pain, or for any illness or condition with which you may suffer, contact one of the organizations listed in *Natural Resources*, page 188, for more information. Next, we'll show you how to use the information we've provided in this book to develop a responsible, comfortable therapeutic plan that can help relieve your back pain.

BACK TIP

Carry with Care

If you must carry heavy objects, hold them close to your body at your waist. Avoid shopping bags for groceries; carrying heavy things at arm's length places undue pressure on the lower back. Instead, package groceries in a paper bag and carry it with both arms.

"It takes a long

time to

become young."

Pablo Picasso

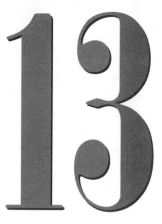

Developing an Alternative Plan

ou've now had a chance to read about the many natural alternatives to surgery and drug therapy available to treat back injuries and back pain. Although some of these options may seem confusing and occasionally contradictory, they all have the same goal in common: to bring your body into a natural state of balance so that your musculoskeletal system can function properly.

Nevertheless, there are significant differences in philosophy between various alternatives. Deciding which alternative is best for you is a highly personal decision, one that may involve investigating several different options before committing to one or another treatment plan.

In the meantime, take a look at the following ideas about how to use and choose an alternative health care method:

1. *Use holistic medicine as a preventive tool.* The best time to explore a new form of treatment is not during a medical crisis, but rather when your body is in a state of relatively good health. It is never too early to make sure that your body is in balance by following a holistic approach to health. By doing so, you may be able to prevent an acute injury or back spasm from occurring as well as avoid stress-related chronic strains and pains over the long-term.

2. *Invest in some bibliotherapy.* A fancy name for learning through reading, bibliotherapy will help you gain a more thorough understanding of the various philosophies of health and disease before you decide how you would like to address your back pain problem. In *Natural Resources*, page 188, you'll find a list of the most relevant books on back pain and natural medicine from which you can choose.

3. *Work with a mainstream physician who is willing to explore options with you.* As we move toward the twenty-first century, more and more medicine is bound to include the best of both mainstream and alternative options. If your physician is willing to learn, but does not know much about these options, you can share your resources, and this book, with him or her. If you are currently being treated by a physician who is not open to other philosophies, you may want to consider choosing another doctor. See Chapter 3 for more information on how to find a doctor you can work with comfortably.

4. *Live well and in harmony with the universe.* If after you've read this book, you decide not to pursue an alternative form of medical care, you still should attempt to open your heart and mind to the natural flow of energy, within and outside of your body. Think about the way you live your life on a day-to-day basis: Is it truly healthy? Does the food you eat nourish your spirit and your body, or do you end up feeling bloated and grouchy? Are you ever able to relax completely, or do you feel under constant pressure? Are your muscles, tendons, and bones strong and supple, or do you often feel stiff, sore, and achy after performing the mildest of exercise? Consider the way you feel every day, and if you think you could feel better, work to make small, incremental changes in your daily habits—even if you decide to forgo a comprehensive natural medicine approach to your back pain problem.

The rest of this chapter is devoted to answering some of the questions my back pain patients have asked me and my colleagues about their specific problem, as well as about the various treatment options described in this book. We hope that the answers provided address some of your own questions and concerns.

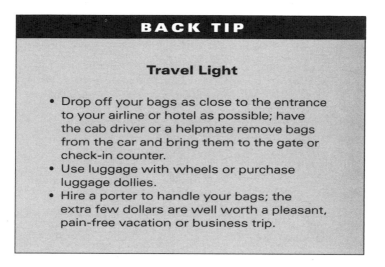

BACK TIP

Travel Light

- Drop off your bags as close to the entrance to your airline or hotel as possible; have the cab driver or a helpmate remove bags from the car and bring them to the gate or check-in counter.
- Use luggage with wheels or purchase luggage dollies.
- Hire a porter to handle your bags; the extra few dollars are well worth a pleasant, pain-free vacation or business trip.

Natural Medicine, Back Pain, and You

Q. Both my father and sister—for whom I have a great deal of respect—are mainstream medical doctors, and I've lived to the age of 42 using mainstream medicine to help me survive a car accident and appendicitis. I know that I'm alive today thanks to the high-tech medical care I received at the hospital after those events. I want to explore alternatives, but I don't want to give up on what has worked for me in the past.

A. There is no doubt that modern medical technology saves lives and can help an individual during an acute crisis. Nevertheless, the effectiveness of modern medicine has its limits, including its typical lack of attention to prevention and its frequent inability to address the root causes of chronic, lifestyle-based conditions like back pain. Fortunately, we are living in a time when high-tech medicine and its holistic counterparts are learning to work in cooperation with one another. Osteopathy is a particularly good example. Osteopaths are medical doctors with access to, and an affinity for, mainstream medical techniques. Many chiropractors, acupuncturists, and other alternative practitioners also have medical degrees and/or working relationships with mainstream doctors and health care facilities. Therefore, you'll still have access to the lifesaving (or pain-reducing) diagnostic and medical therapies you feel work for you while you're investigating holistic options.

Q. I've been suffering with lower backaches almost constantly for about a year. At least once or twice a week, I take a muscle relaxant so that I can sleep, and I practically live on ibuprophen and aspirin. Are there alternative therapies that will allow me to quit taking these drugs?

A. All forms of alterative medicine have at least one goal in common: to allow the body to return to its natural state of balance and health. Medication like aspirin and ibuprofen, on the other hand, works by masking symptoms like pain and discomfort: symptoms that are meant to be warning signs that something has gone wrong in the body. Although pain medication can be enormously helpful in reducing the often agonizing pain of an acute back spasm, these drugs may end up doing you more harm than good if you don't address the underlying cause of your back pain. It makes sense for you to begin to look for other solutions than using these drugs on a daily basis.

Q. I'm very interested in finding a healthy alternative to drugs and surgery and have been reading about the many different options, particularly traditional Chinese medicine. But I've never been a religious person, and the emphasis on a spiritual force that helps us heal bothers me.

A. In one sense, spirituality is a belief that we are connected to and dependent upon something outside of ourselves, whether that something is nature, each other, or the unknown. It is important to distinguish this from a religion, which involves a specific belief system that defines and explains that connection. Although Eastern healing systems stem from philosophical and religious beliefs, it is perfectly possible to derive benefits from these systems without subscribing directly to the encompassing philosophy. What is important is to hold belief that you have the power to control your health and your future, and that you can do this by altering the external world (by diet, stopping smoking, exercising, and changing stressful situations) and the internal world (by not holding onto emotions, by learning to relax, to love, and to play, and by encouraging hope and positive thoughts). Perhaps, through this process, you'll also find a new way to address spirituality in your life.

Back Pain: Assessing Your Risks

Q. My father suffered from back pain and now so do I. Could something like this be hereditary? Should I worry about my kids?

A. Nature versus nurture is one of the oldest conundrums in medicine. It could be that you've learned a muscle or bone weakness or deformity from your father. It is more likely, however, that you inherited from him certain unhealthy habits, such as overeating, underexercising, smoking cigarettes, or leading a life filled with too much stress. With your doctor or natural practitioner, you should explore both possibilities. As for your own children, it's never too early to instill healthy habits that will help your children maintain proper balance and health. By instilling proper diet and exercise habits in your children from a very young age, you could help prevent them—as well as yourself—from developing musculoskeletal problems later in life.

Q. I'm five months pregnant and my back is killing me. Is this normal?

A. You are not alone, far from it. Most pregnant women, at one time or another, suffer from some type of back pain, and for a number of reasons. First, the frequent fatigue and nausea that occur during early pregnancy may discourage a normally active woman from exercising. Second, long periods of bed rest or inactivity can lead to muscle aches and pains. During late pregnancy, the enlarged abdomen may cause the same kind of immobility as well as straining lower back muscles. Follow these hints to find relief:

- Avoid prolonged standing, which encourages painful back arching.
- Avoid prolonged sitting, which places stress on the spine and tends to weaken abdominal muscles.
- Change positions frequently, helping to improve circulation to the muscles and joints of the back and legs.
- Practice the pelvic tilt from both a standing and prone position.

Q. I've been working as a seamstress for a fashion designer for about eight months. I love my job, but my neck and upper back are under constant strain. With exercise, I'm able to work out most of the stiffness, but I'm afraid that, over time and as I get older, the pain will become entrenched. What can I do to keep my job but protect myself from injury?

A. You're right to start thinking about a solution now, before too much damage to your muscles and joints has been done. The first step you might want to take is to consult a specialist in ergonomics: a person trained in making the workplace safe and efficient. He or she will work with you to make sure that your sewing machine is in an optimal position, that you hold your fingers, wrists, and shoulders properly as you sew, and that your seat level is correct. All of these measures will help protect you from injury as you work.

Back Pain: A Medical Overview

Q. What are back pain drugs? Do they work?

A. Man-made drugs, also called pharmaceuticals, are not necessarily considered "bad for you"; in fact, some drugs may be veritable lifesavers under certain circumstances. As discussed earlier, however, pharmaceuticals usually focus on alleviating symptoms, not on addressing underlying problems. They also tend to take over body functions rather than help the body to work properly on its own. Finally, drugs often produce unpleasant side effects that, in essence, only add to the state of imbalance that caused the original symptoms to occur. Choosing more natural approaches, such as dietary measures, exercise, and herbal remedies, that attempt to restore the body to proper working order while producing a minimum of side effects is often a much safer alternative.

Q. Three years ago, I had surgery to repair a herniated disc. Up until about three months ago, it seemed like the operation was a complete success, but now I'm having pain again. My surgeon claims that it isn't uncommon to need a second surgery, but I'd rather not go through it all again. Should I?

A. I would hesitate to give you a definitive answer without first seeing your medical records and examining you. It is possible that surgery could correct your problem. However, whether or not you decide to submit to another procedure, it is imperative that you and your doctor attempt to identify what is causing your discs to herniate. Do you have a job that places great stress on the muscles and joints of your back? Do you drive long distances? Are you completely sedentary? Are you overweight? If you can answer yes to any of these questions, your lifestyle might need as much adjustment as your spine.

Q. I want a homeopath to treat my chronic back pain. My mainstream physician, who admits to being able to offer me few solutions, objects strongly. What should I do?

A. That's a delicate question without an easy answer. Many reputable and highly qualified mainstream physicians find it difficult to accept the tenets of homeopathy and other forms of alternative health care because many haven't been "proven" according to strict mainstream criteria. But as more studies confirm that mainstream medicine can do little for the victims of back pain, more mainstream physicians are willing to explore options with their patients. If your doctor refuses, then I might suggest that you find a new mainstream physician, one who is more willing to explore other treatment options with you.

Exercise: The Path to a Healthy Back

Q. I know that exercise is an important part of any treatment for back pain relief, but I also know that exercise can cause injuries. I also have high blood pressure. Should I exercise or not?

A. Before you start any exercise program, get your doctor's permission. If your back is seriously injured or your blood pressure dangerously high, he or she may recommend very mild and short periods of exercise for a number of weeks—say, walking at a slow pace for ten minutes—until you build up some cardiovascular and muscular endurance. Your doctor will probably recommend that you have a stress test performed at various intervals to test the strength of your heart. However, starting and sticking with an exercise plan will definitely increase your cardiovascular health, and your general sense of well-being, over the long term.

Q. I love to play tennis, and it's about the only exercise I get on a regular basis. But whenever I do an overhead backhand, I seem to wrench my back. What can I do, besides stop playing or losing to an opponent who can spot my weakness?

A. Ask a trained sports therapist to work with you to help identify your problem. The root of the problem might your form: You may be hitting the ball improperly, thereby straining your muscles. Or you might need to strengthen your back, hip, and/or leg muscles through weight training or other exercises before they are strong enough to properly execute the stroke.

Q. I'm a real couch potato, and I want to change my life. But almost every time I start to exercise, I end up throwing my back out. How I can exercise safely?

A. The cardinal rule is to start slowly and build gradually. One of the most frequent and potentially dangerous mistakes people make when they first turn over a new exercise leaf is to push their bodies too hard too quickly. When you next start an exercise program, first ask your doctor or alternative health care practitioner for advice. He or she may have an opinion as to what is causing your back muscles, in particular, to become injured. Then, try to choose an exercise that puts as little strain and pressure on your back and hips as possible, at least until you are stronger and more supple. See Chapter 4 for more information.

Relaxing Out of the Pain

Q. I have a high-pressure job as a criminal defense attorney, and typically work 12 to 14 hours a day. I know I need to relieve some stress—I often suffer from neck pain and backaches and have been known to snap at people—but it seems that every time I try to relax, I only end up getting more tense. How do I resolve this frustrating dilemma?

A. Take a look at the way you're trying to relax. Although we tend to relate inactivity with relaxation, many people find that activities that stimulate their minds and/or bodies—such as exercising or working at a hobby—are more helpful in relieving stress than sedentary, passive activities like watching television or forcing themselves to nap. At the same time, it is important for your general health, as well as for the health of your back, to try to slow down and quiet your mind on a regular basis. A meditation technique like creative visualization which does engage the imagination, may be one way for you to both relax and to get in closer touch with what makes you such a driven and tense person in the first place.

Q. Every night after I get home from work, I spend five or ten minutes writing down everything that I have to do the next day and all the things that are bothering me. I think it helps me relax, but my wife claims that it only makes my problems seem more important than they are. Who's right?

A. More than likely, you are. A study at Pennsylvania State University showed that people were able to reduce their anxiety levels by setting aside a "worry period" every day. If they started to fret about their problems or future tasks at other times in the day, they forced themselves to postpone it until that period. The organization such a system provided gave the subjects a feeling of control that calmed them down. I'd say you were on the right track.

The Diet and Nutrition Factor

Q. I've been dieting since my doctor told me that the excess weight I'm carrying is part of the reason why my lower back hurts so much. I've cut out almost all fat from my diet, mostly because I'm using so many of the fat-free products now available, but I haven't been able to lose any weight. In fact, I think I've gained some. What am I doing wrong?

A. You may be eating as many calories and sugar as you have in the past, or maybe more. Although consuming too much fat, particularly saturated fat like butter and animal fat, is the major cause of weight gain, the fact is that eating too much food of any kind—fat-free or not—will put on the pounds, too. Indeed, every time you eat more calories than you burn off, you gain some weight. Make sure you're not overloading on empty calories—like those that make up fat-free chocolate cake—at the expense of lower-calorie, healthier foods like grains and fresh fruits and vegetables.

Q. I consume quite a lot of diet soda. Could the preservatives and additives in the soda be contributing to my back pain?

A. It's possible that a sensitivity to those substances could be irritating your joints and muscle tissue. However, I would look at more likely sources of your back pain first, such as how much or little you exercise, the work you perform on a daily basis, and your posture, before assuming that an allergy is at the root of your problem.

Q. I'm allergic to pollen; every spring, I wheeze like crazy and my nose runs constantly. I also suffer from back pain, pretty much all year long, but it doesn't seem to be affected by pollen. Could some other allergy be contributing to my back problems?

A. It is true that a person who has an allergy to one substance is more prone to develop another allergic problem. It could be that your immune system is hypersensitive to a certain food or other substance which may be aggravating your muscles and joints. Check with your doctor and/or alternative health care provider.

Q. I love to eat fish and hear that it's a good source of protein and pretty low in fat. Am I right?

A. As long as you don't cook your fish in fat or load it with heavy cream sauces or dressings (like tartar sauce), you've made an excellent choice for your general health and for any weight-loss efforts you've embarked upon. Not only does fish tend to have less fat than meat, but the fat that is in fish contains a special substance, omega-3 fatty acids, which have been shown to reduce the aches and pains associated with inflammation. Fish especially high in omega-3s include salmon, mackerel, herring, sardines, tuna, and anchovies.

Q. Is it possible to cure back pain through diet alone?

A. Because the causes of back pain—indeed, of any chronic disease—are varied and complex, it is unlikely that changing just one aspect of your life will permanently alleviate your back pain problems. Keeping yourself at a normal weight and providing your body with all the raw materials it needs to build and maintain muscle and bone will, of course, help you stay balanced and centered. Bringing your body into a true state of harmony involves addressing nutritional deficiencies or excesses, as well as examining your emotional and spiritual state and working to find inner peace. That's why a holistic approach, as embodied in traditional Chinese or Indian medicine, is a good choice for many people suffering from chronic back pain.

Hands-On Help: Bodywork and Massage

Q. After an unpleasant experience with Rolfing, which I found too painful, I've been hesitant to try other bodywork techniques. At the same time, I know that my posture is out of kilter, which is part of the reason I suffer from so much lower-back pain. Is there another program that might help me?

A. Although Rolfing can be quite effective, it is not a painless method of manipulating the spine and joints. Many people with back pain enjoy the slow, controlled, and gentle changes in posture that result from practicing the Alexander technique. Reread Chapter 7 and explore *Natural Resources*, page 188, for more information.

Q. Much to my surprise, my back pain was greatly relieved by a massage therapist who concentrated, not on my back, but on my feet. What's the connection?

A. It sounds as if your therapist is familiar with the concept of "trigger points," or pockets of injured tissue in one part of the body that can cause pain in a distant site, even in your back. Remember, your body works as a unit, and whenever one part of it is injured, another part may well be affected. By massaging your feet, your therapist is helping to heal injured tissue in your feet that may have been referring pain to your back for years.

Spinal Manipulation: Chiropractic and Osteopathy

Q. Can spinal manipulation, with all of the cracking and pressing it involves, end up hurting rather than healing my back?

A. When performed by a trained professional, spinal manipulation will not damage the joints or muscles of the back. In fact, the idea is to bring your spine back into its proper alignment and thus relieve aches and pains that occur when your body is out of position. And keep in mind that some of the cracking and popping you hear occurs when gasses are released from inside the joints when they are moved.

Q. I've been seeing a chiropractor for a lower-back injury and my doctor has told me that my blood pressure, which had been on the high side, is now normal. Could there be a connection?

A. Absolutely. Depending on where on the spine your chiropractor is working to alleviate your lower-back problems, therapy may be helping to reduce your blood pressure in one of two ways. If your chiropractor is concentrating on your neck area, it's likely that he or she is helping to balance the activity of the sympathetic and parasympathetic nervous systems in the function of the heart and blood vessels. The midback area, on the other hand, is connected to kidney function; it is likely that your kidney is producing more urine or the adrenal glands, which sit atop the kidney, are producing a hormone that helps to lower blood pressure.

Q. What kind of training does a chiropractor usually have?

A. To be certified as a chiropractor, an individual studies at a chiropractic college for a minimum of four years. Training includes all of the basic science and diagnostic skills taught to a medical student, but does not involve surgical or pharmaceutical study. Some chiropractors also learn the fundamentals of nutrition as well.

Chinese Medicine and Back Pain

Q. I'm deathly afraid of needles, but I'm ready to try anything that might help relieve my chronic back pain. My brother goes to a traditional Chinese medicine practitioner whom he trusts. Should I put my fears aside and go too?

A. Before you decide upon acupuncture, talk to your health care practitioner about your anxiety. There are many other options within traditional Chinese medicine, including acupressure, massage, herbal treatments, and dietary measures, that you might want to consider.

Q. I have been to an acupuncturist who used a lot of needles, and left them in for a long time. My friend went to another acupuncturist who used very few needles, and just stuck them in and out. What is the difference?

A. There are several different systems of acupuncture being practiced in the United States, depending on the acupuncturist's training. Chinese-style acupuncture, as you experienced, tends to use several needles which are retained for several seconds or minutes. Japanese style uses a more gentle stimulation and fewer needles, and French style, favored by many physician-acupuncturists, is somewhere in between. English five-element style tends to focus on the relationship of emotions to the symptoms, while some others tend to address specific physical symptoms. It is best to discuss the system with the acupuncturist prior to or at the first appointment.

Q. I would try acupuncture, but I'm worried about AIDS. Is this a risk with acupuncture needles?

A. In this era of AIDS awareness, it is highly likely that your acupuncturist is using disposable, single-use acupuncture needles. In addition, all licensed acupuncturists are required to take clean-needle training as part of their examination for licensure. Even so, it is important to ask your prospective acupuncturist if he or she uses disposable needles.

Ayurveda: Medicine from India

Q. I was surprised to learn that enemas are frequently prescribed to treat back pain in Ayurvedic medicine. What's the relationship?

A. According to Ayurvedic theory, most back pain is caused by an imbalance of *vata*—one of the three primary forms of energy in the body, and the main site of *vata* is the colon. Along with dietary restrictions, massage therapy, and herbal prescriptions, enemas help to cleanse the body and thus bring *vata* back into balance.

Q. Ayurvedic medicine seems very elaborate and multilayered. How much do I have to understand before I can start to heal my back pain and bring my body back into balance so that I don't reinjure myself?

A. Learning about your body from an Ayurvedic perspective is a process that may take many years, indeed a lifetime. An Ayurvedic practitioner will guide you through that process while providing you with practical information about proper diet, exercise, herbal medicine, and meditation techniques. If you follow this advice, you should see a positive change in the state of your health relatively quickly, probably within a period of several weeks, depending on your condition.

Q. I don't have a lot of time during the day to both exercise and meditate. Can I do both at the same time with yoga?

A. Yes. Yoga is used as both a form of exercise and a method of attaining a higher state of consciousness through proper breathing and meditation. The beauty of yoga exercise lies in its ability to bring the body into balance through quiet, powerful stretching and the spirit into a more relaxed state through focused breathing and, sometimes, creative visualization.

The Healing Power of Herbs and Aromas

Q. I'm interested in treating my chronic back pain with herbs. But I also take medication for an ulcer. Can herbs interfere with the drugs I'm taking?

A. Herbs *are* drugs, and yes, if your physician and herbalist do not work together—or are at least aware of how each is treating you—you could run into some problems with the effectiveness of your treatment plan. It's up to you to supply all the people who treat you with a list of any and all medications and remedies you are taking.

Q. Is aromatherapy only used for relaxation or do the herbs from which oils are derived have physical effects as well?

A. First of all, it's important to realize that relaxation *is* physical. Remember, more and more evidence is surfacing every day that emotions—and thus the effects of emotion—are present in every cell of your body, including those of your muscles, tendons, ligaments, and bone. Second, there is some evidence that therapeutic particles of the original plants enter the body through the nasal passages and the skin and work internally the same way a dose of herbal medicine by mouth would work.

Q. I'm allergic to penicillin and a variety of antibiotics. Could I be allergic to herbal remedies as well?

A. Absolutely. And you must be sure to inform your herbalist of any and all allergies and sensitivities you may have to drugs and other substances. This information will help him or her provide you with a safe, effective herbal remedy.

Homeopathy and Back Pain

Q. I visited a homeopath for the first time last week. After asking me lots of questions about my diet and other health problems, he decided to treat my back pain with *Rhus tox*. I understand that this herb comes from the poison ivy plant. I'm quite allergic to poison ivy. Is this dangerous for me?

A. The amount of toxic substance in the homeopathic solution is quite minuscule and thus unlikely to provoke a serious allergic reaction. However, please make sure that the homeopath is aware of your allergy and keep close watch on your symptoms and side effects.

Q. I'm not sure I understand the way homeopathy works, and what I do know makes me unsure that it really does work, but I have friends who swear by it. Do I have to believe in it for the therapy to work?

A. Having faith that a treatment has the potential to work is certainly helpful, but it is not necessary for you to fully understand homeopathy to reap its benefits. In fact, many homeopaths are unsure themselves exactly how a substance diluted so many times still has the power to heal. Nevertheless, millions of people around the world find relief from a variety of ailments with homeopathy and you may be able to do so as well.

In the next section, we describe some of the vast resources available to you in your quest for a safer, more effective, and longer-lasting approach to relieving your back pain and bringing your whole body and spirit into a more balanced state.

Natural Resources

....

$\mathcal{B}$ack pain poses special problems for the modern medical world, problems that mainstream technology appears unable to solve, at least at this point. Fortunately, alternative medicine is becoming more accessible—and more accepted—by more Americans every day. Following is a list of associations and organizations that provide information on all aspects of their respective field, from providing lists of qualified practitioners to explaining their approaches to health and disease. Books, pamphlets, and videotapes are often available, sometimes at no cost, sometimes with a fee. In addition, we have provided a brief bibliography listing some of the hundreds of new and older books that you can read to find out more about all aspects of alternative medicine. Knowledge *is* power: Use these resources to help you to find a solution to back pain that works for you.

Acupuncture/Chinese Medicine

National Oriental Medicine and Acupuncture Alliance
   (Non-physicians)
638 Prospect Avenue
Hartford, CT 06105
(203)232-4825

American Academy of Medical Acupuncture (Physicians)
5820 Wilshire Boulevard, Suite 500
Los Angeles, CA 90036
(800)521-AAMA

National Commission for the Certification of Acupuncturists
1424 16th St. NW
Washington, DC 20036
(202)232-1404

American Foundation of Traditional Chinese Medicine
505 Beach Street
San Francisco, CA 94133
(415)776-0502

Qigong Institute/East-West Academy of Healing Arts
450 Sutter Street
San Francisco, CA 94108
(415)788-2227

READING LIST

Beinfeld, Harriet, and Korngold, Efrem. *Between Heaven and
   Earth: A Guide to Chinese Medicine.* New York: Ballantine
   Books, 1991.

Kaptchuk, Ted. *The Web That Has No Weaver: Understanding
   Chinese Medicine.* New York: Congdon and Weed, 1992.

Liu, Y. *The Essential Book of Traditional Chinese Medicine,
   Vols. 1 and 2.* New York: Columbia Unversity Press, 1988.

Aromatherapy

The Pacific Institute of Aromatherapy
P.O. Box 6842
San Rafael, CA 94903
(415)479-9121

National Association for Holistic Aromatherapy
P.O. Box 17622
Boulder, CO 80308
(303)258-3791

Aromatherapy Institute of Research
P.O. Box 6842
San Rafael, CA 94903

Lotus Light
P.O. Box 1008
Wilmot, WI 53170
(414)889-8501

READING LIST

Hymann, Daniele. *Aromatherapy: The Complete Guide to Plant and Flower Essences*. New York: Bantam Books, 1991.

Lavabre, Marcel. *Aromatherapy Workbook*. Rochester, VT: Healing Arts Press, 1990.

Rose, Jeanne. *The Aromatherapy Book*. Berkeley, CA: North Atlantic Books, 1992.

Ayurvedic Medicine

Ayurvedic Institute—Dr. Vasant Lad
11311 Menaul NE Suite A
Albuquerque, NM 87112
(505)291-9698

American School of Ayurvedic Sciences
10025 NE 4th Street
Bellevue, WA 98004
(206)453-8022

The College of Maharishi
Ayurveda Health Center
P.O. Box 282
Fairfield, IA 5256
(515)472-5866

READING LIST

Chopra, Deepak, M.D. *Ageless Body, Timeless Mind.* New
York: Harmony Books, 1993. *Perfect Health,* 1991.
Quantum Healing, 1990.

David, O.M.D. *Ayurvedic Healing.* Salt Lake City: Morson Publishing, 1990.

Heyn, Birgit. *Ayurveda: The Indian Art of Natural Medicine
and Life Extension.* Rochester, Vermont: Healing Arts Press,
1983.

Back Pain

American Academy of Orthopedic Surgeons
222 South Prospect Ave.
Park Ridge, IL 60068
(708) 823-7168

American Chronic Pain Institute
P.O. Box 850
Rocklin, CA 95677

National Chronic Pain Outreach Association
7979 Old Georgetown Rd., Suite 100
Bethesda, MD 20814
(301) 652-4948

North American Spine Association
222 S. Prospect Avenue #127
Park Ridge, IL 60068
(708) 698-1628

READING LIST

Abraham, Edward A., M.D. *Freedom from Back Pain: An Ortho-pedist's Self-Help Guide.* Emmaus, PA: Rodale Press, 1986.

Benjamin, Ben E., Ph.D. *Listen to Your Pain.* New York: Penguin Books, 1984.

Bresler, David E. *Free Yourself from Pain.* Topanga, CA: The Bresler Center, 1992.

Fine, Judylaine. *Conquering Back Pain: A Comprehensive Guide.* New York: Prentice-Hall Press, 1987.

Hall, Hamilton. *The Back Doctor.* New York: McGraw-Hill, 1980.

Harold, D.M.D. *Pain Without Prescription.* New York: Harper Perennial, 1982.

Klein, Arthur C., and Sobel, Dava. *Backache Relief.* New York: Penguin Books, 1986.

Prudden, Bonnie. *Pain Erasure.* New York: M. Evans and Co., 1980.

Sarno, John, M.D. *Mind Over Back Pain.* New York: Berkeley Books, 1986.

White, Augustus A., M.D. *Your Aching Back.* New York: Fireside Books, 1990.

Biofeedback

Association for Applied Psychophysiology and Biofeedback
10200 West 44th Avenue, Suite 304
Wheat Ridge, CO 80033
(303)422-8436

Center for Applied Psychophysiology
Menninger Clinic
P.O. Box 829
Topeka, KS 66601
(913)273-7500

READING LIST

Danskin, David G. and Crow, Mark. *Biofeedback: An Introduction and Guide.* Palo Alto, CA: Mayfield Publishing Co., 1981.

Bodywork and Massage

North American Society of Teachers of the Alexander Technique
P.O. Box 3992
Champaign, Illinois 61826
(217) 359-3529

Feldenkrais Guild
P.O. Box 489
Albany, Oregon 97321
(503) 926-0981

The Rolf Institute
P.O. Box 1868
Boulder, Colorado 80306
(303) 449-5903

Zero Balancing Association
P.O. Box 1727
Capitola, CA 95010
(408)476-0665

READING LIST

Barlow, Wilfred. *The Alexander Technique*. New York: Alfred Knopf, 1973

Feldenkrais, Moshe. *Awareness Through Movement*. New York: Harper & Row, 1977.

Prudden, Bonnie. *Myotherapy: Complete Guide to Pain-Free Living*. New York: Ballantine Books, 1984.

Rolf, Ida. *Rolfing: The Integration of Human Structures*. New York: Harper & Row, 1977.

Smith, Fritz. *Inner Bridges*. Atlanta: Humanics, Ltd., 1994.

Chiropractic and Osteopathy

American Chiropractic Association
1701 Clarendon Boulevard
Arlington, VA 22209
(703)276-8800

International Chiropractors Association
1110 North Glebe Road, Suite 1000
Arlington, VA 22201
(703)528-5000

World Chiropractic Alliance
2950 N. Dobson Road, Suite 1
Chandler, AZ 85224
(800)347-1011

READING LIST

Coplan-Griffiths, Michael. *Dynamic Chiropractic Today: The Complete and Authoritative Guide to This Major Therapy.* San Francisco: HarperCollins, 1991.

Palmer, Daniel David. *The Chiropractor's Adjuster.* Davenport, IA: Palmer College Press, 1992.

Diet and Nutrition

American College of Nutrition
722 Robert E. Lee Drive
Wilmington, North Carolina 28480
(919)452-1222

American College of Advancement in Medicine
P.O. Box 3427
Laguna Hills, CA 92654
(714)583-7666

READING LIST

Braverman, Eric R., M.D. and Pfeiffer, Carl C., M.D. *The Healing Nutrients Within*. New Canaan, CT: Keats Publishing, Inc., 1987.

Hass, Elson M., M.D. *Staying Healthy with Nutrition*. Berkeley, CA: Celestial Arts Publishing, 1992.

Lappe, Frances Moore. *Diet for a Small Planet*. New York: Ballantine, 1982.

Herbal Medicine

American Association of Naturopathic Physicians
2366 Eastlake Avenue, Suite 322
Seattle, WA 98102
(206)323-7610

The American Herbalists Guild
P.O. Box 1683
Sequel, CA 95073

The Natural Apothecary
169 Massachusetts Avenue
Arlington, MA 02174
(617)641-1378

Herb Research Foundation
1007 Pearl Street, Suite 200
Boulder, CO 80302
(800) 748-2617

READING LIST

Castleman, Michael. *The Healing Herbs*. Emmaus, PA: Rodale
Press, 1991.

Hoffman, David. *The Herbal Handbook*. Rochester, VT: Healing Arts Press, 1987.

Kowalchick, Claire and Hylton, William, editors. *Rodale's Illustrated Encyclopedia of Herbs*. Emmaus, PA: Rodale Press,
1987.

Murray, Michael. *The Healing Power of Herbs*. Rockin, CA:
Prima, 1992.

Homeopathy

Homeopathic Educational Services
2124 Kittredge Street
Berkeley, CA 94704
(800)359-9051

International Foundation for Homeopathy
2366 Eastlake Avenue
Seattle, WA 98102
(206)324-8230

National Center for Homeopathy
801 North Fairfax
Alexandria, VA 22314
(703)548-7790

READING LIST

Cummings, Stephen, M.D. *Everybody's Guide to Homeopathic Medicines*. Los Angeles: Jeremy P. Tarcher, Inc., 1991.

Lockie, Andrew. *The Family Guide to Homeopathy*. New York: Prentice-Hall Press, 1993.

Ullman, Dana. *Discovering Homeopathy: Medicine for the 21st Century*. North Atlantic Books, 1991.

Meditation and Mind/Body Medicine

Institute of Transpersonal Psychology
P.O. Box 4437
Stanford, CA 94305
(415)327-2066

Mind-Body Clinic
New England Deaconess Hospital
Harvard Medical School
185 Pilgrim Road
Cambridge, MA 02215
(617)632-9530

Stress Reduction Clinic
University of Massachusetts Medical Center
55 Lake Avenue, North
Worcester, MA 01655
(508)856-2656

The Center for Mind-Body Studies
5225 Connecticut Avenue NW
Washington, DC 20015
(202)966-7388

READING LIST

Benson, Herbert. *The Relaxation Response.* New York: Outlet Books, Inc., 1993.

Borysendo, Joan. *Mending the Body, Mending the Mind.* New York: Bantam Books, 1988.

Kabat-Zinn, Jon. *Full Catastrophe Living.* New York: Delta Press, 1990.

Locke, Steven, and Colligan, Douglas. *The Healer Within.* New York: Mentor, 1986.

Moyers, Bill. *Healing and the Mind.* New York: Doubleday, 1993.

Yoga

Himalayan Institute of Yoga, Science, and Philosophy
RRI Box 400
Honesdale, PA 18431
(800)822-4547

International Association of Yoga Therapists
109 Hillside Avenue
Mill Valley, CA 94941
(415)383-4587

READING LIST

Hewitt, James. *The Complete Yoga Book*. New York: Schocken
Books, 1977.

Monro, Robin, M.D., et. al. *Yoga for Common Ailments*. New
York: Fireside Books, 1990.

Alternative Medicine/General Reading

Goldberg Group (350 physicians). *Alternative Medicine: The Definitive Guide*. Puyallap, WA: Future Medicine Publishing, Inc., 1993.

Monte, Tom, and editors of "EastWest Natural Health." *World Medicine: The East West Guide to Healing Your Body*. New York: Tarcher/Perigree, 1993.

Murray, Michael, and Pizzorno, Joseph. *Encyclopedia of Natural Medicine*. Rocklin, CA: Prima Publishing, 1991.

Words and Terms to Remember

....

Active movement: Normal range of voluntary movement of a joint.

Acupoints: Acupuncture points throughout the body which correspond to specific organs.

Acupressure: A healing art based on the fundamentals of Chinese medicine in which finger pressure is applied to specific sensitive points on the body.

Acupuncture: A technique used in Chinese medicine that involves the insertion of small needles under the skin to activate the flow of energy within the body.

Aerobic exercise: Physical exercise that relies on oxygen for energy production.

Alexander technique: A technique concerned with improving posture to reduce or prevent back pain.

Allopathy: Term for standard Western medicine; from the Greek *allos* (different) and *pathein* (disease, suffering), thus implying the use of drugs whose effects are different from those of the disease being treated.

Anaerobic exercise: Exercise that draws upon the muscles' own stores of energy and does not require oxygen, such as weight-lifting and isometric exercises.

Analgesic: A drug that relieves pain, including aspirin, Darvon, and codeine.

Ankylosing spondylitis: An inflammatory disease of the spine that causes pain and fusion of the bony part of the spine.

Anti-inflammatory agents: Drugs designed to reduce swelling, inflammation, and pain. Some common antiinflammatory drugs include Feldene (piroxicam), Motrin (ibuprofen), and Voltaren (diclofenac sodium).

Arthritis: Inflammation and irritation of the joints.

Articulation: The place of union, or junction, between two bones.

Autonomic nervous system: The part of the nervous system responsible for bodily functions such as the heartbeat, blood pressure, and digestion. It is divided into two divisions, the sympathetic nervous system and the parasympathetic nervous system.

Biofeedback: A behavior modification therapy in which patients are taught to control bodily functions such as blood pressure through conscious effort.

Carbohydrate: Organic compounds of carbon, hydrogen, and oxygen, which include starches, cellulose, and sugars, and are an important source of energy. All carbohydrates are eventually broken down in the body to glucose, a simple sugar.

Cauda: The terminal portion of the spinal cord.

Central nervous system: The brain and the spinal cord, which are responsible for the integration of all neurological functions.

Cervical spine: The portion of the spinal column in the neck region composed of seven vertebrae.

Channels: Also called meridians. In traditional Chinese medicine, the invisible pathways of qi on the surface of and within the body.

Chinese medicine: A philosophy and methodology of health and medicine developed in ancient China.

Coccyx: The structure at the very tip of the spine, connected to the bottom of the sacrum, made up of about three or four fused vertebrae; also called the tailbone.

Connective tissue: Highly vascular tissue that forms the supporting and connecting structure of the body.

CT scan: A computerized tomogram (x-ray image) that can be reconstituted by a computer to depict bone and soft tissues in several planes.

Deficient condition: In traditional Chinese medicine, a disorder resulting from the body's inability to maintain equilibrium.

Detoxification: In Ayurveda, the process of removing toxins from the body.

Disc: Fibrous tissue with an inner core of gelatinlike material located between adjoining spinal vertebrae and serving a shock-absorbing function.

Disc degeneration: The loss of the structural and functional integrity of the disc, which may or may not cause pain.

Doshas: In Ayurvedic medicine, the three basic forces of energy which determine an individual's balance and body type.

Endorphins: Natural substances produced by the body which function as natural painkillers.

Epinephrine: Also called adrenaline. A hormone secreted by the adrenal glands that increases the heart rate and constricts blood vessels.

Essential oil: Concentrated, pure aromatic essence extracted from plants.

Excess condition: In traditional Chinese medicine, a condition in which qi, blood, or body fluids are disordered and accumulate in channels or elsewhere in the body.

Extension: Backward bending of the spine.

Facet joints: Located behind the vertebral body, these paired joints connect the posterior elements of the vertebrae. They permit the spinal bones to glide over each other when the back is in motion.

Fascia: A sheet or band of connective tissue that separates various muscles and organs within the body.

Fight-or-flight response: The body's response to perceived danger or stress, involving the release of hormones and subsequent rise in heart rate, blood pressure, and muscle tension.

Flexion: Bending forward of the spine.

Fracture: An injury to a bone in which the tissue of the bone is broken.

Gluteus: Muscle of the buttocks.

Hamstring: The large muscle located at the back of the thigh.

Herniated disc: Displacement of disc components beyond the normal confines of the annulus, the outer fibrous portion of the intervertebral disc.

Holistic: Pertaining to the whole body; treatment of disease by taking into consideration every part of the body to bring the internal environment into balance.

Homeopathic remedy: A remedy, selected on the basis of the similarity of its symptoms, that produces a reaction in a patient that leads to a cure.

Law of Similars: The principle of "like shall be cured by like," which forms the basis of homeopathy; the proper remedy for a patient's disease is that substance that is capable of producing, in a healthy person, symptoms similar to those from which the patient suffers.

Ligament: A strong, elastic band that holds a joint together and that, in the spine, keeps vertebrae in place by supporting and strengthening discs and vertebral joints.

Limbic system: A group of brain structures that influence the endocrine and autonomic motor systems.

Lumbar spine: The five weight-bearing vertebrae located between the thoracic vertebrae and the sacrum; also known as the lower back.

Lumbosacral sprain: An injury to the muscles, ligaments, and/or tendons of the lumbosacral (lower-back) region.

Manipulation: Technique used in chiropractic therapy to adjust the spine, joints, and other tissue.

Meridians: In traditional Chinese medicine, the fourteen channels in the body through which the energy known as qi runs.

Mobilization: A technique of chiropractic therapy that gently increases the range of movement of a joint.

Moxa: Dried mugwort leaves used in traditional Chinese medicine; placed on the end of needles then lighted and held near an acupuncture point to warm and tonify qi.

Muscle spasms: Involuntary, painful contractions of muscles.

Musculoskeletal system: The muscles and skeleton.

Myelogram: A radiological test in which the spinal cord, nerves, nerve roots, and surrounding space can be visualized.

Neurological deficit: Loss of reflexes and/or normal motor strength.

Neurotransmitters: Substances that transmit messages to, from, and within the brain and other body tissues.

Nicotine: The addictive chemical substance derived from tobacco that affects blood pressure and brain activity.

Norepinephrine: A hormone secreted by the adrenal gland in the "fight-or-flight response" that raises blood pressure and acts to stimulate muscle contraction.

Obesity: The condition of excess fat accumulation in the body, usually considered present when a person is 20 percent above the recommended weight for his or her height and age.

Osteopathy: A branch of Western medicine that focuses primarily on the manipulation of the musculoskeletal system while taking a holistic approach to health.

Osteoporosis: A condition in which the bones of the body lose minerals and thus become weak and porous.

Palpation: Physical examination of the body using the hands to feel for abnormalities.

Parasympathetic nervous system: The division of the nervous system that, when stimulated, slows heart rate, lowers blood pressure, and slows breathing.

Pelvic tilt: The body position in which the abdominal muscles are contracted and the buttocks tucked down and under the spine.

Pitta: An Ayurvedic dosha.

Potency: The dilution of homeopathic remedies to increase their effectiveness, thus giving them their therapeutic value.

Qi: In traditional Chinese medicine, the life force or energy of the body, and the universe, that circulates through the body's channels.

Qi stagnation: Any blockage of energy in the body that interrupts the body's natural functions or the healing process.

Quadriceps: The muscles located in the front of the thighs.

Risk factor: Condition or behavior that increases one's likelihood of developing a disease or injury.

Rolfing: A massage technique that focuses on realigning the fascia—the connective tissue that envelops the muscles and organs. The goal of rolfing is structural integrity, or making sure that all of the organs, bones, and tissues are properly positioned within the body.

Sacrum: The portion of the spine below the lumbar region.

Sciatic nerve: The largest nerve in the body, located in the hip region and extending down the back of each thigh to the knee.

Scoliosis: A congenital misalignment of the spine in which the spine curves sideways.

Shen: In traditional Chinese medicine, the "spirit" or consciousness, which both originates and forms the outward expression of human life.

Shiatsu: A massage technique developed in Japan and based on the Chinese medical philosophy that believes that disease and pain are caused by blocked qi (energy) in energy pathways in the body. By applying pressure to the blocked meridian, relief from pain and disease may result.

Spinal column: The column of individual bones (the vertebrae) that surround and protect the spinal cord and support the back.

Spinal cord: A network of nerve fibers that relay messages and sensations to and from the brain, running from the base of the skull through the open portion of each vertebrae.

Spinal fusion: A surgical procedure using bone grafts to connect two or more vertebrae.

Spondylosis: Abnormal bone fusion of a vertebral joint; general term for degenerative changes in the spine.

Stress: Any factor, physical or emotional, that threatens the health of the body or otherwise requires a response or change.

Subluxation: In chiropractic, a term used to explain a misalignment of spinal vertebrae.

Succussion: The forceful shaking of liquid homeopathic remedies that allows the permeation of the original substance into the alcohol tincture.

Sympathetic nervous system: The division of the autonomic nervous system responsible for such functions as blood pressure, salivation, and digestion; works in conjunction with the parasympathetic nervous system.

Symptoms: Observable or internal changes in the mental, emotional, and physical condition of a person; in holistic medicine, symptoms are the external proof of an internal imbalance.

Tao: The course of nature and ways of nature; a Chinese term denoting the universe as an undifferentiated whole.

Tendon: The connective fibers attaching the muscles to bones; when a muscle contracts, or shortens, it pulls on the tendon, which moves the bone.

Thoracic: The twelve vertebrae of the spine in the mid and upper back where the ribs attach to the spine.

Tincture: An alcoholic solution of a medicinal substance.

Tonify: In Chinese medicine, to nourish, augment, and invigorate; to add to the supply of qi and to promote the proper functioning and balance in the body.

Toxin: Substance that is harmful or poisonous to the body.

Trapezius: Muscle of the upper back.

Vata: An Ayurvedic dosha.

Vertebrae: The bones that form the spine or backbone, permitting the erect stance, flexibility, and mobility of the body.

Vital force: In homeopathy, the intangible energy that animates all living creatures and mediates their physical, emotional, and intellectual responses to external stress.

Yang organs: In Chinese medicine, the yang organs are hollow or surface organs such as the intestines, spleen, gallbladder, and skin.

Yin organs: In Chinese medicine, the yin organs are dense, internal organs such as the heart, liver, lungs, kidneys, and bones.

Yin/yang: Chinese concept that describes all existence in terms of states or conditions that are different but mutually dependent; traditional Chinese medicine aims to restore balance to these contrasting aspects of the body and mind.

Index

....

About the Authors

....

Glenn S. Rothfeld, M.D.

Glenn S. Rothfeld, M.D., is founder and Medical Director of Spectrum Medical Arts in Arlington, Massachusetts, a comprehensive primary care center blending orthodox and complementary medical styles. He holds one of the nation's first Master's Degrees in acupuncture, and is director of the Western Medical Curriculum at the New England School of Acupuncture. He is also Clinical Instructor at Tufts University School of Medicine, where he teaches a popular course in Natural Medicine.

Suzanne LeVert

Suzanne LeVert is a writer who specializes in health and medical subjects. Her recent titles include A Woman Doctor's Guide to Menopause, Parkinson's Disease: A Complete Guide for Patients and Caregivers, *and* If It Runs in the Family: Hypertension and Diabetes. *She lives in Boston, Massachusetts.*